The Cult and Science of Public Health

The Cult and Science of Public Health

A Sociological Investigation

Kevin Dew

Berghahn Books
New York • Oxford

Published in 2012 by

Berghahn Books
www.berghahnbooks.com

Library of Congress Cataloging-in-Publication Data

Dew, Kevin. The cult and science of public health : a sociological investigation / Kevin Dew.
p. cm. Includes bibliographical references and index.
ISBN 978-0-85745-339-6 (hardback : alk. paper) – ISBN 978-0-85745-340-2 (ebook)
1. Public health–Social aspects. 2. Medical policy. 3. Health services accessibility. 4. Health attitudes. I. Title.
RA418.D493 2012 362.1–dc23

2011041094

British Library Cataloguing in Publication Data

A catalogue record for this book is available from the British Library

Printed in the United States on acid-free paper

ISBN 978-0-85745-339-6 (hardback)
ISBN 978-0-85745-340-2 (ebook)

Contents

Acknowledgements

Although I am responsible for the arguments made in this book I am indebted to the many people who have engaged with me in research, teaching and scholarship over the years. I would particularly like to thank John Gardner for all the work he did in helping to shape many of the chapters in this book, and Sarah Donovan for casting an editorial eye over many of the chapters. A special thank you to students whom I have supervised and whose work has introduced me to new ways of thinking and challenged my preconceptions, in particular Penelope Carroll, Monika Clark-Grill, Vivienne Ivory, Mondy Jera, Joanna MacDonald, Jennifer Martin, Anna Matheson, Kathy Nelson, Chrissy Severinsen and George Thomson.

Much of the material in this book draws on research and publications with a number of colleagues. I would like to acknowledge and thank past and present members of the Applied Research on Communication in Health (ARCH) group in this regard, particularly Maria Stubbe, Tony Dowell, Lindsay Macdonald, Rachel Tester and Libby Plumridge. Other important collaborators on research, supervision and writing related to this book have included Ginny Baker, Tony Blakely, Donna Cormac, Jackie Cumming, Ruth Fitzgerald, Simon Hales, Sarah Hill, Philippa Howden-Chapman, Vera Keefe-Ormsby, Allison Kirkman, Mike Lloyd, Tom Love, George Major, Eileen McKinlay, Deborah McLeod, Losa Moata'ane, Bridget Robson, Tim Rochford, Louise Signal, Dave Slaney, Keitha Small, Katrina Taupo, Sonya White and Alistair Woodward.

The Department of Public Health at the University of Otago, Wellington, provided me with much food for thought in relation to public health, and I would like to thank all the members of that department for being such fantastic colleagues over many years. The Sociology and Social Policy Programme at Victoria University of Wellington is my current academic home, and colleagues here have provided an excellent environment for writing and sharing ideas.

Over the last decade or so I have been generously supported in my research by different funding agencies and this research has informed the development of my ideas. I would particularly like to acknowledge the Health Research Council of New Zealand, the Marsden Fund and the Lotteries Commission. I would also like to thank the journals which have published papers that include material that this book draws on, and the many reviewers who have so often enhanced my writing and helped to hone my interpretations. Finally, I would like to thank Jody Orgias, and Hedley and Nathan Dew, for being such wonderful people to be with, for keeping my feet on the ground, and for allowing me the time and space to write this book.

INTRODUCTION
Public Health Theories and Theorizing Public Health

Introduction

What we can eat, what hazards we face at work, what diseases we should immunize our children against, how we should respond to the health impacts of climate change, where we should smoke and drink alcohol, what is placed in the water we drink, what impact income redistribution policies have on health – these and a great deal else besides are the province of public health. Public health is a collective response to threats against people's health (Eberhart-Phillips 1999). It can be divided into two major phases. What is called 'the old public health' primarily concerned itself with health protection and disease prevention. Such concerns related to issues of water quality, sewerage disposal, food quality, and the use of vaccinations. The new public health has not replaced the old public health, but has added on concerns for health promotion and health development (Beaglehole 1992). This is a more educative function, where stress is placed on individual responsibilities for health and the idea of empowerment, so that people are able to make informed choices about health. New public health may also emphasize ecological principles that can take into account broader conditions of living such as the state of the urban environment and sustainable development (Knight 1999). It can also focus on the social determinants of health – those particular features of society, such as the state of the housing stock, the level of discrimination and inequality in a society, protective measures taken in the workplace and much else besides, that impact upon our life chances.

As public health initiatives involve collective action or treatments that affect the population it is a thoroughly social and political enterprise. Many issues in public health lead to disputes and controversies. Debates are had over the fluoridation of the water supply, the introduction of new vaccines to established vaccine schedules, the relationship between pharmaceutical companies and the World Health Organization (WHO), and the efficacy and value of mass screening programmes for such diseases as prostate cancer. The stance we take on these issues may relate to any number of factors, such as whether commercial or vested interests are involved, our faith in experts and science, or the political acceptability of a particular initiative. Views on how individual rights should be balanced against the public good are central to debates about public health. As such, public health is an immensely rich and intriguing discipline to view from a sociological perspective.

Public health can mean many different things and act in many different settings. It can mean healthy school dinners, community-level neighbourhood renewal, marsh drainage, sewerage systems, public transport and cultural revivals. Public health concerns can take in global trade, the natural environment, the built environment, the local economy, the community and lifestyle (Orme et al. 2007b: 671). The public health workforce includes public health physicians, environmental health officers, public health nurses, youth workers, health promotion specialists, and a range of others whose work incorporates elements of public health, such as teachers and social workers (Barrett et al. 2007).

As an academic discipline, public health has some intriguing elements. Besides attempting to understand the relationships between health and society, many public health researchers see themselves as advocates, and have strong links with policy development. For many, public health is about a commitment to change (Orme et al. 2007a). From this perspective public health is not conservative; it is not preserving the status quo. It is transformational and utopian in vision. Public health advocates may, for example, envisage a society where there is no inequality in health outcomes.

Public health draws on a vast array of disciplines, including sociology, psychology and demography in the social sciences, biology and physiology and the myriad of sub-disciplines in the natural sciences, and a range of interdisciplinary entities such as urban planning and resource management. One uniting concept of the diverse institutional spaces of public health is a focus on the population, and not the individual (Orme et al. 2007b). In terms of official pronouncements, public health was defined in 1988 by Donald Acheson, Chief Medical Officer for England, as 'the science and art of preventing disease, prolonging life and promoting health through the organized efforts of society' (Acheson, cited ibid.: 13). Although the first medical officer of health was appointed in Britain in 1847, it was not until 1972 that public health medicine became formally recognized within the medical profession in the U.K. with the establishment of the Faculty of Public Health (ibid.). This is suggestive of the marginal status that public health has had within the profession of medicine itself.

The focus of public health has changed over the modern period, and within public health today we can see a number of different orientations to the objectives of public health and the values underpinning the discipline. The sanitation movement in the nineteenth century has a particular focus on infectious diseases. In the mid-twentieth century, risk factor epidemiology developed which was oriented to chronic disease and a 'downstream' focus on lifestyle factors. In the latter part of the twentieth century the sub-discipline of social epidemiology came into its own with its focus on the social determinants of disease – looking 'upstream' at issues of housing, employment and social organization more generally.

Public Health Foundation Stories

Foundation stories are important. They tell us something of the values and aspirations of institutions, disciplines, organizations and nation-states that invoke them. We can consider two quite distinct public health foundation stories. One is of John Snow and the Broad Street pump, the other is of Rudolf Virchow and Prussian mining communities.

The John Snow story is elaborated upon in chapter 1. This foundation story of modern public health dates back to 1854 when Dr John Snow removed the handle of the Broad Street drinking-water pump in London as he had hypothesized that the water from this pump was the cause of a cholera epidemic. This is a story of the foundations of epidemiology, which is the study of diseases and their causes at a population level, and also of the role of public health in bringing about change. The story is illustrative of the core values of public health – rational science and passionate advocacy (Green 2008). Not only did Snow identify the cause of disease via an epidemiological strategy, but he took action to prevent it by removing the pump handle. This supports the definition of public health that includes a commitment to change, based on rational, scientific principles.

The Rudolf Virchow story has a slightly different flavour. We can see the John Snow story as a technical solution to a disease problem uncovered by the workings of science. Virchow, at a very similar time to Snow, 1848, studied a typhoid epidemic in Prussia. He studied it by living with the miners and their families in the areas afflicted by the epidemic. He noted that these families were affected by many other diseases, and that the reason for this lay in their social condition. These families suffered from poor housing, poor working conditions and a poor diet. The solution to this situation was not a simple technical one, but required a transformation in the way society was organized. It required better wages, education, food production and progressive tax reform (Green and Labonté 2008b).

In these two examples we can see quite different approaches to public health. Both aimed to improve the health of the population, and both required collective effort to bring about change. But the Snow version, as received, was a collective effort to identify the causes of disease and provide the resources to bring about some improvement. The status quo at the economic and political level could be maintained. But even here there is a hint of something more radical in that the whole society was responsible for protecting all citizens from disease – and so the ideas of individual responsibility and laissez-faire or free-market politics are subject to critical analysis. But the Virchow version of public health was radical to its roots – calling for fundamental change and social justice.

The vision of public health has been articulated in different ways. Reducing human suffering is one aspect, but creating the conditions of human health is another (Zierler and Krieger 2008). Public health researchers and practitioners can draw upon a variety of frameworks to orient their practices. These include biomedical and lifestyle frameworks, but also feminist, political economy, human rights and ecosocial frameworks (ibid.). For example, the drug economy of the U.S. and the social and political forces that brought about that economy can be seen as important variables explaining the increase in HIV among poor black and Hispanic American women (ibid.). Racism, gender inequalities, and the outcomes of a particular form of capitalist production, are salient features in explaining such a situation.

The radical and critical element in public health is not marginal to the discipline. The journal *Radical Community Medicine* clearly expressed this stance in its title, which continued with its name change to *Critical Public Health*. The Virchovian values can now be seen as part of mainstream public health (Green and Labonté 2008a). Such a critical element raises concerns about the determinants of the determinants – that is, what are the conditions that give rise to the particular distributions of the current social determinants of health? What powers are at play? How can we facilitate social justice and overcome health inequality? In the words of Green and Labonté, 'Critical public health is not a disinterested academic discipline, but one that engages with structures of power to challenge as well as describe them' (ibid.: 4). Such an enterprise is partisan and adversarial.

The 'new' public health, which was coined as a concept in the latter part of the twentieth century, called for a renewed focus on social and economic determinants of health in contrast to the curative services more commonly associated with health care (Green and Labonté 2008a). A watershed in the development of the new public health was WHO's *Ottawa Charter for Health* of 1986 (ibid.). In this charter, the prerequisites of health were articulated as including social justice and equity, sustainable resources, education, income and peace. Health promotion was then the province of all sectors in society, not just public health (World Health Organization 1986). Unequal health outcomes are a particular problem to be remedied in this version of the new public health.

Within the particular discipline of social epidemiology there has been debate about the specific causal pathways that lead to health inequalities. Social epidemiology rejects the notion that the causal pathways can simply be related to genetics or individual choice, and claims that there is something about the relationship between the social world and the biological world that helps explain disparities in health outcomes. Social epidemiology has been described as 'a marriage of sociological frameworks to epidemiological inquiry' (Krieger 2001: 669). Although the term social epidemiology appeared for the first time in an article in *American Sociological Review* in 1950, it was not until the end of the twentieth century that the first textbook with that term appeared (ibid.). Social epidemiology has proffered a number of theories to explain the different patterns of disease in populations (ibid.). These could be captured in three overarching positions – the materialist, psychosocial and ecosocial positions.

The materialist argument, very closely related to the social production of disease argument, suggests that unequal access to material factors such as good nutrition, decent housing, health care, and the socially organized production and distribution of health hazards has the major impact on the health of individuals. The unequal access to resources and unequal exposure to health hazards points to political processes as a root cause of health inequalities, whether those political processes are politicized, developed and articulated at a national level that foster free markets, or international policies imposing structural adjustment programmes on nation-states. The free market, or unhindered capitalism, exacerbates social, and therefore health, inequalities.

The political economy perspective challenges current capitalist processes including those that foster uneven economic development (Whiteis 2008). Dramatic and disturbing figures describing the unequal distribution of wealth as a variable explaining health inequalities are highlighted, such as that less than 25 per cent of the planet's population live in industrialized countries but these countries have over 80 per cent of global GNP, that poor debtor countries in the south remit billions of dollars a month in interest repayments alone to the rich north, or that the infant mortality rate in developed countries is around 6 per thousand whereas in developing countries the rate averages 200 per thousand (Larkin 2008). In the U.S. the top 1 per cent of households experienced a 17 per cent gain in real net worth between 1983 and 1995 whilst the poorest 40 per cent suffered an 80 per cent decline in net worth (Whiteis 2008). Poverty is associated with the most prevalent mortalities and morbidities, such as postnatal infectious diseases, lead poisoning and violence (ibid.). With economic segregation paralleling racial segregation, higher mortality rates are experienced by minority and indigenous groups. U.S. black mortality rates are over 50 per cent higher than the rates for whites (ibid.).

Economic differences alone do not account for differences in mortality rates between ethnic groups (Tobias et al. 2009). In addition to political economy approaches and the explicit focus on unequal access to resources, public health research has also described and theorized the impact of colonization on indigenous peoples. For almost every measure of morbidity and mortality, indigenous peoples fare worse than the colonizers and their descendents (Labonté 2008). In Australia, the gap in life expectancy between indigenes and settlers is as much as 21 years, and in the U.S. it is 4–5 years (ibid.). Indigenous peoples have been forced into the market economy through displacement from traditional sources of food as traditional land has been altered or taken in the name of economic development (Lambert and Wenzel 2008). In this context, diseases of poverty have been called diseases of colonization and racism, where colonization and racism mean the experience and consequences of poverty are different for indigenes and settlers (Robson 2008). For example, an indigenous person in poverty is likely to be exposed to poverty for longer, have fewer assets, have less choice in relation to housing, be more likely to come under the surveillance of the police, and so on (ibid.).

In contrast to the materialist position, the psychosocial position emphasizes the stresses that rigid social hierarchies can have in damaging health. In this view, both physical and psychological stress explain the observation that there are differences in people's susceptibility to disease (Krieger 2001). Psychological stress can lie in rigid hierarchies, but also rapid social change, marginal social status and traumatic social events such as bereavement (ibid.). Terms such as social capital and social cohesion have been deployed within this approach to public health – the focus being on the support networks available in social settings that provide greater resilience to disease for some people.

The psychosocial argument has been given credence from a famous research programme studying the stress effects of hierarchy, known as the Whitehall study (Brunner and Marmot 1999). This programme studied seventeen thousand British civil servants. It found that there was a relationship between the employment grade in the civil service and health-related psychosocial factors. These factors included low control over work, a lack of variety in work, and a lack of social contact. The researchers found that there were metabolic changes associated with a person's position in the workplace hierarchy, including changes in blood glucose levels and blood-clotting mechanisms. The research supports the view that long-term exposure to psychosocial stresses in the workplace may lead to increased risk of conditions such as heart disease and diabetes. Although these studies have been limited to workplaces, the mechanisms affecting health could apply to the general population. The psychosocial argument has led to discussion of the influence of social hierarchy and the implication that relative inequality (not just absolute inequality, where material factors are most influential) might affect health outcomes.

Ecosocial theories attempt to encompass both materialist and psychosocial positions. They foster, as Krieger (2001) states, an 'analysis of current and changing population patterns of health, disease and well-being in relation to each level of biological, ecological and social organization'. This analysis can go from the cell through to the ecosystem. Proponents argue that it includes the materialist or social production of disease perspective, but links this to biology. In explaining racial differences in the experience of health conditions, the psychosocial focus on stress can be included, alongside analyses of institutional discrimination, disparities in socio-economic status and the biological impact of economic deprivation (ibid.). There is an attempt to integrate across all these levels.

More recently, in exploring public health interventions, there has been an interest in the contribution that complexity theory can make. Complexity theory developed out of the sciences of mathematics, biology and physics and has increasingly been articulated as a theory to explain the behaviour of non-linear systems in the social sciences. It promotes a non-linear view of causality, with interrelationships between systems and within systems (social, ecological, political, economic systems and so forth) being a central focus for understanding causal processes, and has specifically been applied to public health interventions (Matheson et al. 2009).

In sum, public health theorizing is as diverse as the disciplinary foundations of public health. Understandings of causality will undoubtedly continue to change, drawing on the ideas of other disciplines, with some particular perspectives being foregrounded at times while others recede into the background. The relationship between public health understandings and the environment have also changed over time. In chapter 1 we will see the early development of public health with its focus on the urban environment and its links to disease. In the twentieth century there was an increasing focus on non-communicable diseases, like lung cancer and heart disease, which shifted the focus from the environment to the individual in terms of explanations for outcomes and interventions to improve health. But in the latter part of that century a renewed focus on the social and economic determinants of health brought the environment back into focus (Green 2008). The development of concerns around environmental change has considerably changed the focus again, and newer developments have attempted to integrate the social and the biological.

Sociological Positions on Public Health

The argument made in this book is that a Durkheimian perspective can provide insights into the place of public health in contemporary society. Public health researchers have been influenced by Durkheimian theorizing in a number of ways, in particular the concept of anomie developed in his book *Suicide* (for example Rhoades 2003), and also more indirectly with the deployment of the concept of social capital in relation to the integrative mechanisms in communities (Razzell and Spence 2005; Whitley and McKenzie 2005). It is suggested here that there are other valuable concepts articulated by Durkheim, such as those found in his discussions on the role of religion in society, that can be drawn on to understand public health. An organizing concept for this book is considering public health as a religion in Durkheimian terms. A religion of modern society, as predicted by Durkheim, is variously called a cult of humanity, of man, of the personality and of the individual. The cult of humanity is the term preferred here. An argument is put forward that public health may function as the cult of humanity.

For Durkheim, in modern society a cult of humanity would perform the roles and functions of traditional religion in premodern society. This is not a cult in the popular sense. It does not involve brainwashing or conspiracy. It is, for Durkheim, a social institution like other religions, and Durkheim refers to religions as religious cults. The increasing division of labour and social differentiation in modern society requires a different form of religion. This new religion or cult of humanity would express the unity of society and would centre on our humanity – the one thing we hold in common in a highly differentiated society. This cult then could be seen as a humanist religion. It would be based on rationality and science, but would have a function that science alone is unable to perform – to act as a force of moral regulation. For Durkheim, new forms of moral regulation are required in modern society in order to constrain the anomic desiring that would be a consequence if social institutions did not provide a check on individuals. This new religion would emphasize social justice and sympathy for human suffering.

This book is not an examination of theories about the causation of the patterns of population health but an examination of the role that public health plays in contemporary society, and an argument is made that public health in contemporary society can usefully be seen in terms of a moral force that functions like religious forces did in earlier societies.

In the analysis of public health itself and the way it can be conceptualized in contemporary society, Durkheimian concepts have not been explicitly drawn on. Sociologists and others who have analysed public health have tended to draw on conflict or collectivist perspectives and Foucauldian influenced analyses.

Conflict analyses in sociology align with public health materialist or political economy theories of causation, and are influenced by Marxist analyses. This approach focuses on power held by different groups or classes in society, the material influences on health and disease, the impact of production on disease, and the unequal distribution of public health resources that favour those who are privileged and disadvantage the poor. The latter is most famously captured in the concept of the inverse care law, which states that the availability of medical care varies inversely with the need for medical care in the population (Tudor Hart 2000). That is, the poor, who suffer a higher burden of illness, use fewer health care and medical resources than those who are more advantaged. From a conflict perspective public health, as part of medicine, could be conceptualized as 'an ideological expression of class domination' where 'medicine is revealed as an ideology stabilizing the power of the state and society's other established authorities' (Gerhardt 1989: 254). Feminist orientations to public health have varied and have included critiques of public health for focusing on diseases of middle-aged white men (Inhorn and Whittle 2001). Feminist perspectives have also exposed the tension between public health and the feminist movement in relation to screening campaigns (Hyde 2000; Willis 1999). Such analyses have leant themselves to critiquing health promotion programmes that focus on changing individual behaviours (Fox 1993).

Foucauldian analyses have been more explicitly concerned with an examination of the ontological status of disease and health. As will be further discussed in chapter 3, Foucault argued that one important dimension of the power over life that has been evolving since the seventeenth century is that of a biopolitics of the population that focuses on biological processes that become subject to regulatory controls (Foucault 1988). In this vein, Armstrong argues that the rise of surveillance medicine in the twentieth century was based on the problematization of the normal, in that it 'brings everyone within its network of visibility' (1995: 395). A notion of 'precarious normality' positions few as truly healthy and everyone as open to surveillance, calculations of risk, and intervention. Much of the focus here has been on the relationship between discourses and practices (Lupton 1994). In this framing, public health is one disciplinary technique that 'inveigles itself into our lives and identities' regulating our bodies and rendering us docile (Ryan 2005: 17). Petersen and Lupton encapsulate this position when they state that '[u]nder the imperatives of public health, personal/individual and public welfare are one and the same' (1996: 88). Coercive methods forcing conformity may still exist, but these have largely been replaced by self-regulation. Knowledge and power are inseparable, so as knowledge and understandings change, new forms of power emerge. From this perspective the discipline of sociology itself no longer offers an oppositional stance (as it might from a conflict perspective where it could focus on the social causes of disease) but is an aspect of medicalization itself (Gerhardt 1989).

Postmodern perspectives critique the totalizing procedures of public health and health promotion, and seek to resist them by focusing on choice, otherness and difference, most notably captured in Nicholas Fox's concept of arche-health (Fox 1993). Such a perspective is founded on the notion that terms such as health and illness are no more and no less than discourses without any ontological basis (ibid.). These discourses have a constraining and moral purpose, and one that must be resisted in order to achieve an authentic ethical-political involvement in health.

Both the collectivist and Foucauldian-inspired analyses of the function of public health position the institution as negative and demanding resistance, either to combat and overcome social inequity or to lay claim to authenticity. A Durkheimian reading positions public health differently.

Durkheim has been presented in much sociological literature as a functionalist. However, Taylor and Ashworth (1987: 39) argue that 'Whereas functionalists sought to explain relationships between observable parts of a social system, Durkheim was concerned with structures that lie behind observable phenomena'. In other words, Durkheim is positioned here as a realist. The social facts that Durkheim was concerned with in such works as *Suicide* and *The Elementary Forms of Religious Life* were sources of moral authority in society (ibid.).

For Durkheim there are four contradictory moral forces in society, described as altruism (a commitment to a higher order outside of the self), egoism (individuality), fatalism (inescapable limits to human action) and anomie (uncertainty, change). Modern society is characterized as one that has high levels of egoism and anomie (Taylor and Ashworth 1987). Without social mechanisms to constrain egoism and anomie, pathological consequences – such as suicide – will follow. These social mechanisms would then need to promote altruism, and possibly fatalism. Durkheim looked to a number of possible sources to constrain egoism and anomie such as occupational groupings. Another constraining force is found in religion, which in contemporary society takes the form of a cult of humanity.

Considering public health in terms of a contemporary religion is not to claim that public health is an irrational discipline. Durkheim suggested that this cult of humanity would have to be based on science and subject to the critical elements of science (Durkheim 1915). But the social practice of religion would also go beyond science, as science is always incomplete and the social practices of science do not unite society in a collective fashion.

Durkheim argued that the historical growth of the state was a cause of the rise of the cult of humanity or the cult of the individual, and that 'the stronger the State, the more the individual is respected' (from *Leçons de Sociologie: Physique Des Moeurs et du Droit* cited in Lukes 1973: 270). More rights would be granted to the oppressed (Mestrovic 1991). The state was also:

> A special organ whose responsibility it is to work out certain representations which hold good for the collectivity. These representations are distinguished from the other collective representations by their higher degree of consciousness and reflection. (Durkheim 1957: 50)

For Durkheim the state had an important moral role in society:

> It is not merely a matter of increasing the exchanges of goods and services, but of seeing that they are done by rules that are more just; it is not simply that everyone should have access to rich supplies of food and drink. Rather, it is that each one should be treated as he deserves, each be freed from an unjust and humiliating tutelage, and that, in holding to his fellows and his group, a man should not sacrifice his individuality. And the agency of which this special responsibility lies is the State. (Durkheim 1957: 72)

On the other hand, Durkheim was very concerned about the possibility of an inflated state that could develop into the 'veritable sociological monstrosity' of absolutism (cited in Ramp 2003: 124).

So the cult of humanity is born from the state, but it is argued here that public health, as a cult of humanity, has an ambivalent relationship to the state. It can play a role in tempering the 'monstrous' tendencies of the state, but can also, at particular historical moments, play a role in facilitating the monstrous state. These tensions will be explored in the following chapters.

Green and Labonté argue that public health has always been marginal in policy and the academy (2008a). This may be the case, but the argument made in this book views public health, in its many forms, as an increasingly pervasive influence on social organization and social formations, even if individual practitioners of public health may have less status than their surgical and consultant medical colleagues.

Taking the view that public health fits as a cult of humanity within a Durkheimian framework provides public health advocates and academics with a way of integrating their own roles in relation to the politics and science of population health. The following chapters in this book will demonstrate how it allows for an exploration of the negative aspects of the moral constraints associated with the discourses of public health and health promotion, but also the positive functional aspects, and the way in which public health as an institution provides a means of resistance to dominant discourses in contemporary society around consumption and neo-liberal notions of freedom.

This book is not a survey or description of public health, but it provides an argument about the place of public health in contemporary society. Public health is an important moral force, and as such plays a significant role in mediating between different institutions, including the state and the market. But like all institutions, it too needs to be tempered and mediated, lest it shape society in its own image.

CHAPTER 1
Myths, Morality and Modern Public Health

Introduction

In German states in the eighteenth century, national policies and public health became closely entwined in the development of the 'medical police' (Rosen 1993). The medical police were state bureaucrats whose goal was the regulation of all aspects of human activity to foster the health of the nation. It was, as Rosen puts it, a form of enlightened despotism: all spheres of human activity, even the most private of individual affairs, were to be regulated for the benefit of the state. Johann Peter Frank, a leading advocate of medical policing, lobbied for bachelor taxes to encourage marriage, and for legislation that would enforce periods of rest for new mothers. The mothering and education of children were to be under police supervision, and Frank also prescribed in great detail the necessary diet, clothing, sanitation and recreation required to produce a population of healthy individuals. The goal of medical policing was to regulate health practices from the womb to the tomb through a systematic and comprehensive health policy (Rosen 1993: 164). Importantly, the justification for such measures was to improve the health of the state as a whole, and it was to this end that individual health was important.

The concept of medical police openly acknowledges the relationship between social control and public health. In order to bring about communal changes in health, individual freedoms may have to be limited, and non-conformists punished. Similar measures were adopted in other parts of the world: a course on medical police appeared in the Edinburgh medical school curriculum in 1809 (Smith 2007) and the policing of climate, physical education, and medicine were advocated. The Metropolis Management Act 1855 made the appointment of 'inspectors of nuisances' compulsory in London – and these inspectors were known as the medical police. In some jurisdictions the medical police's powers included prosecuting for obscene language (Wood 2005). They had the powers to enter premises and even comment on domestic spaces such as the positioning of privies in houses (ibid.). In the eighteenth century their roles could include occupational hygiene and administration of hospitals, but by the nineteenth century this narrowed down to the control of epidemic diseases, the oversight of environmental sanitation and the implementation of sanitary surveillance.

This concern with the health of individuals so that the state itself is empowered has been a recurrent issue in public health up to the present day, yet is not a prominent feature of what have become its 'founding myths'. This chapter will begin with a brief overview of such myths, which tend to focus mostly on public health's discovery of scientific principles and commitment to individual well-being. This chapter will then go on to show, however, that the development of public health reveals that, unsurprisingly, it has been far more complex and riddled with conflict and tensions than such myths would indicate. There was in many cases a reluctance to adopt public health measures, either because there was doubt about their efficacy, or it conflicted with prevailing ideologies. When public health measures have been adopted, it has often been for reasons that cannot be reduced to paternalistic benevolence. As public health has developed, it has constantly brought about novel social and material relations. These have presented new, often unpredicted challenges and prospects for action. This chapter demonstrates some of the ways in which public health can come into conflict with business enterprise and with the general public. Drawing on a Durkheimian framing we can see how public health can act to restrain the state, particularly in relation to its free market ideologies, and restrain the individual.

As noted in the introduction, the foundation story of modern public health and epidemiology dates back to 1854 when Dr John Snow hypothesized that a cholera outbreak in London was caused by drinking water contaminated by sewage. John Snow's 'study' has been hailed as 'a model of the scientific, investigative approach to medical research, and clearly identified water as the medium by which the disease was transmitted' (Halliday 2007: 77). In this story, John Snow marked on a map of London where all the deaths from the cholera outbreak had occurred. From this he identified the particular area of trouble and developed his theory about the cause of the outbreak. To prove his theory he removed the handle of the Broad Street pump where the contaminated water was coming from, and so the epidemic disappeared (Brody et al. 2000). The power of this story for public health lies in a number of factors. John Snow believed that cholera was caused by some organism in contaminated water, a theory that we now accept but which was hotly contested at the time. Current theories of cholera identify faeces-contaminated water as the means of spread, along with flies that have hatched in diseased faeces (Halliday 2007). But in the early 1800s, speculation about the cause of such diseases as cholera was rife. *The Lancet* noted that people had escaped a cholera epidemic 'by rubbing their bodies with a liniment containing wine, vinegar, camphor powder, mustard, pepper, garlic and ground beetles' (ibid.: 59). There were theories that cholera was the result of an emanation from the earth, from atmospheric electricity or from a shortage of ozone. A commonly held theory, articulated by Justus von Liebig, Professor of Organic Chemistry at the University of Giessen, was known as the zymotic theory. This theory posited that disease was the result of the putrefaction of organic material giving rise to contagious miasmas that spread infection through breathing (Halliday 2007). This became better known as the miasmatic theory of disease, and it was believed that foul odours, bad air, or a noxious atmospheric influence could be the source of a miasma and cause disease.

Miasmatic theories of disease causation were popular in the nineteenth century, and were at odds with the germ theory being promoted by Snow. Snow's actions showed that this miasmatic theory was incorrect. His achievement is thus held as embodying the progressive nature of public health. Rather than being driven by theory, Snow simply applied a method of careful observation that drew him to the logical conclusion – the same conclusion anyone would come to if they followed the same logic. In addition, Snow is seen as being a founder of epidemiology, the study of patterns of disease and their causes.

There are many elements of this story of John Snow that have been contested by medical historians. Snow did not derive his theory from what he had found in his map, but drew his map to illustrate the prior theory that he had been working on for many years. In other words, he drew the map to support his theory, and made various editions of the map with changes in detail, such as altering the political boundary lines to highlight the areas where deaths occurred (Brody et al. 2000). Choices in representation were made to support an argument. Snow himself did not remove the handle, but after his report on the epidemic to the Board of Guardians of St James Parish, where the Broad Street pump was located, the handle was removed. Despite this, the story suggests that public health and epidemiology are not driven by theories, but by observation. Another important element of this story is that it shows that public health is about engaging in action. To paraphrase a famous saying by Karl Marx and apply it to public health, public health is not only about understanding the world, but changing it. John Snow did not simply locate the source of the problem; he sought to ameliorate it by removing the pump handle.

More recently, John Snow has come to be framed as a founder of community engagement. The story goes that during the epidemic there was one person affected by cholera that did not live in Broadgate, but lived in an affluent area some distance away. Snow found out from this person's maid that she drank the water from the Broad Street pump because it was sweeter. Consequently, Snow's detective work and active involvement is held as being the origin of the public health physician's engagement with 'ordinary people to find out about their habits and practices' (Orme et al. 2007b: 11).

Logical argument, empirical observation, community engagement and action are then seen as the heart of public health. In the foundation story of John Snow these can be opposed to superstition, tradition, ideology and mere description or analysis of the world. In more recent and contemporary times, public health advocates have focused on the various success stories of public health, particularly the eradication of infectious disease.

Public health measures have been credited with some remarkable achievements. Vaccination is extolled for bringing about a dramatic decline in mortality rates for diseases such as measles, diphtheria, whooping cough and tuberculosis, which in the late nineteenth and early twentieth centuries caused many deaths. Public health vaccination campaigns, along with the use of antibiotics to fight bacterial infections, were deemed to be so successful that it was claimed that as a cause of death, infectious diseases have been reduced to insignificance (Davis 1981). Such claims were obviously made before the emergence of HIV/AIDS.

From this perspective, the fall in death rates from infectious diseases can be seen as an outstanding success in public health. However, apart from smallpox and polio, infectious diseases were well into their decline before vaccines were developed for these diseases. Whooping cough was a disease that could kill hundreds or thousands of people during an epidemic, but from the early 1900s epidemics would rarely cause death. Measles caused severe mortality in 'developed' countries, even through the interwar years, but since then it has been a relatively mild disease (Maclean 1964).

Thomas Mckeown has provided a challenging and provocative argument in relation to this decline. He has argued that medical science was not responsible for the major decline in death rates from infectious diseases that occurred in the late nineteenth and early twentieth centuries. Improved diet and a rising standard of living were responsible for improving resistance to these diseases and so lowering the death rates. The only real exceptions here, Mckeown argues, are vaccinations for smallpox and sanitary improvements reducing the impact of diseases such as cholera and typhoid (Hardy 2001). Otherwise direct human intervention accounted for little in the way of influence on measles, scarlet fever, whooping cough and many other diseases. Vaccines for these diseases were not available when the remarkable drop in death rates occurred, and a vaccine was never developed for scarlet fever. Mckeown's thesis has subsequently been contested – and others have argued that public health interventions have had a greater role in reducing death rates and improving health than Mckeown claims (ibid.).

However, while what accounted for the rapid decline in morbidity from infectious diseases is not absolutely clear, changes in sanitation and sewerage measures and nutritional changes would have had a major part to play in this (McKeown 1979; Szreter 1995). Improvement in the health of children or changes in the virulence of the disease were also seen as possible explanations (Maclean 1964). It should be noted however, that even with the reduction in death rates during the late 1800s, health gains in terms of morbidity were small (Hardy 2001). Health experience was dominated by 'the miserable run of chronic respiratory, rheumatic and digestive illness' (ibid.: 46).

The reality of public health, then, has not been as clear and logical as the picture that is often presented. But these foundation myths persist as important elements in the moral authority that public health exercises in contemporary society.

Modern Developments in Public Health

Early precedents of public health can be found in ancient Greece. In around 400 BCE, the medical discipline of hygiene was developed. In the name of the goddess Hygieia, this discipline 'attempted to control every aspect of the human environment – air, diet, sleep, work, exercise, the evacuations, passions of the mind' (Smith 2007: 74). Hygieia is a concept which conceptualizes health in terms of a perfect human body set within a perfect environment – a wholesome life extending the lives of patients under Greek physicians (ibid.). Perfection was not found in extremes, but in moderation and a balance of opposites (ibid.).[1]

The Protestant Reformation ushered in other views about the care of the body, with diet and cleanliness again being central and a continuing Greek influence leading to the strong promotion of exercise (Smith 2007). The 'reformed body' was kept pure not only through religious practices and demeanour but also through diet (ibid.). Exercise and fitness, however, particularly in relation to sports, was not always an important part of the health and care of the body. While physical prowess, strength, and fitness were prized by the Greeks, sports and games were repressed during the Old Commonwealth in England. These were revived in the Restoration, and in 1724 George Cheyne, the author of the best-selling *Essay on Health and Long Life*, insisted that exercise should be part of a patient's religion (ibid.). This relation between physical and moral health was a popular theme within Christian movements. The Christian mission has historically been associated with helping the poor and indigent, as well as with the mission of healing. William Buchan, the author of the best-selling British health manual – *Domestic Medicine* – published in 1769, wrote: 'There cannot be a more noble, or more god-like action, than to minister to the wants of our fellow creatures in distress ... to instil into their minds some just ideas of importance of proper food, fresh air, cleanliness, and other pieces of regiment necessary in diseases, would be a work of great merit' (cited in Smith 2007: 255).

It is around this time that Johann Peter Frank was advocating the establishment of medical police in the German-speaking states. The view was emerging that population health was vital to the health of the state as a whole: a healthy, fit population of men and fertile, healthy women create a strong, productive and competitive state. For the next two hundred years or so, this was to become a strong argument for adopting public health measures.

George Rosen argued that the development of medical police was symptomatic of a centralized and despotic form of governance common to the German-speaking states. In contrast, medical police would be in conflict with the more laissez-faire approach to governance of eighteenth- and nineteenth-century Britain (Rosen 1993). In comparison with the German-speaking states, the development of public health in Britain was characterized by a great deal of tension with commercial interests. On one hand, there was anxiety that any centralized form of public health would infringe upon the liberal tradition and the individual, and the commercial rights it championed. On the other hand, there was considerable disquiet over the appalling living conditions of a large section of British society.

These appalling living conditions were in part a result of the rapid urbanization that accompanied the industrial revolution. The industrial revolution brought about a spectacular growth in urban centres, with London experiencing a six-fold increase in the population (Halliday 2007). During the nineteenth century the growth of cities and the impacts of industrialization led to shifts in thinking about responsibility for health. It was no longer considered a wholly private matter, but now increasingly regarded as requiring government action (Hardy 2001). This was clearly seen in the development of compulsory vaccination legislation, but also in the increasing use of epidemiology to describe national disease pictures and encourage public health interventions. Prior to the Public Health Act of England and Wales in 1848 governments had responded to public health issues by using decrees, whereby in response to epidemic diseases beds could be burnt, houses fumigated, towns whitewashed and so on.

In England in the late 1800s towns were not kind to human health: 'Their skies were black with coal smoke, their streets strewn with horse manure; in summer they were alive with flies, in winter dank and damp with fog' (Hardy 2001: 13). Sickness at this time came at a great cost. It has been estimated that 72 per cent of pauperism in England in 1871 was the result of sickness (Hardy 2001). For those who found themselves destitute the poor laws ensured that their experience was not a pleasant one, with recipients of poor relief being subjected to the harsh conditions of the workhouses, being politically disenfranchised and forfeiting 'their normal rights as citizens' (Sturdy 2002a: 243). In 1871 the Poor Law Board was abolished and a Local Government Board took over its function. This change heralded a shift from focusing on the poor law as a deterrent to receiving relief to a view that there was a public responsibility to provide medical services (ibid.). Research on the impact of poverty on health supported this change of focus. Charles Booth, a Liverpool shipowner, initiated his research into poverty in London in the 1880s, producing a 'poverty map' to illustrate the levels of deprivation suffered in different areas of the city (Halliday 2007). He concluded, to his dismay, that more than a third of the population lived in poverty (Hardy 2001). Similarly, Seebohm Rowntree, a Quaker industrialist, concluded that a third of York's population lived in poverty and that the working classes received 25 per cent less than the necessary nutritional requirements for physical efficiency (Hardy 2001).

Many families in nineteenth-century Britain became reliant upon state relief measures after the male breadwinner died from acute infectious disease. Inadequate sewerage systems and water supplies were identified as possible causes for this state of affairs and therefore legislation was developed to deal with the problem (Hamlin and Sheard 1998). An added bonus to governments of introducing public health legislation was that such action might help to quell a working class that was becoming increasingly revolutionary. In addition to impoverished food, harsh working conditions, polluted waterways, poor sewerage systems, and industrial pollution and smog, city dwellers in the 1800s had to cope with an immense amount of animal traffic as they were brought to slaughter houses and markets. Cities had to deal with tons of animal droppings (Halliday 2007).

In 1836 the General Register Office (GRO) was established in the United Kingdom and this has been identified as a crucial development in providing an evidence-base and was an ongoing feature of public health discourse (Mooney 2008). This office provided for the registration of births, marriages and deaths, and more importantly from a public health perspective, the causes of deaths. Such an office provided the foundation for epidemiological studies that could have a profound impact on the development of social and health policy. Although there has been much debate over how best to use summary health measures over time, for example crude death rates, standardized death rates, or life expectancies, measures of this type have been consistently used from the mid-1800s to today (ibid.). Initially they could be exploited to provoke public health and policy action to improve the health of the population, and in turn could be used as a measure of progress in such interventions as sanitary reform (ibid.).

Early examination of this register revealed that 15 per cent of children did not survive to their first birthday in the nineteenth century (Halliday 2007). GRO data showed that Britain was also a divided nation in terms of the experience of health and premature death. Those in the south and in rural areas had lower death and illness rates than those in the north and in the cities (Hardy 2001). In addition, there was a difference in these experiences by social class – a finding that is as notable today.

GRO data provided important information on patterns of death and disease. At the same time some features of urban life came into focus, such as housing conditions. Poor housing was becoming the centre of public health debates. Heavy Irish immigration to Liverpool following the 1845 potato famine meant that it was not unusual to find up to sixty people sharing a four-room dwelling (Halliday 2007). During the late 1800s programmes of slum clearance were common in the major cities and legislation was introduced to improve housing conditions. But medical officers of health were conscious that to enforce such acts would merely shift the housing problem from one district to another. In 1847 Dr William Henry Duncan was appointed as Britain's first medical officer of health in the city of Liverpool (Halliday 2007). The medical officer was to 'inspect and report periodically on the sanatory [*sic*] condition of the said Borough, to ascertain the existence of Diseases, more especially Epidemics increasing the Rates of Mortality' (cited ibid.: 104). The appointment followed campaigns from Duncan and others, which included highlighting the different ages of death in rural and urban areas. In rural areas the average age of death was 36.5 years whereas in the urban areas it was only 19.5 years. Poor sanitary conditions were blamed – such as the 20 per cent of the working population who lived in cellars that were often deep in sewage (ibid.). In the 1890s research undertaken by the medical officer of health of London County Council clearly showed an association between overcrowding and mortality (ibid.). Housing concerns are still alive and well today – but in 1911 in England as much as one-fifth of the population was estimated to live in overcrowded accommodation (Hardy 2001).

The shift towards the adoption of public health and improving housing quality faced considerable difficulties, as illustrated by the following quotation taken from *The Lancet* in 1899:

> It is not an uncommon thing for a Medical Officer, while endeavouring to have some insanitary property put in a proper state of repair, to find that a quantity of it is owned by a member of the sanitary authority – i.e. by one of his masters, by one of the men who have absolute power to discharge him neck and crop. (Cited in Halliday 2007: 24)

Aristocrats and landowners were able to put pressure on local authorities to resist public health measures that could harm their interests – such as efforts to prevent fertilization with sewage in city boundaries for fear of miasmas (Brunton 2002).

On the other hand, there were commercial imperatives fostering quarantine (Smith 2007). Quarantine, a measure first used in the city of Dubrovnik in 1377, was increasingly used to limit the spread of leprosy and the plague. This measure emerged for trade reasons in early modern Italian city-states. By 1500 most major towns in Italy had established health boards that could impose quarantine as well as impose other measures like banning the movement of goods from entering or leaving the town (Nutton 2006). In the seventeenth and eighteenth centuries pan-European regulations were adopted for commercial reasons (Smith 2007). The relationship between public health and commerce was determined by the kinds of impact such interventions would have on trade.

As with resistance to housing interventions there was resistance to efforts to curb city pollution. Clear blue skies were seen as a sign of recession and so laws to curb or limit the outpourings of soot from factories were resisted by workers and manufacturers (Luckin 2002). Governments were also reluctant to act to impinge upon the practices of industrialists – so a light approach was taken to industrial hygiene. As late as 1952 it was estimated that 'the Great Smog' of London killed twelve thousand people, and this event finally prompted the Clean Air Act of 1956 (Halliday 2007). A permissive approach was also taken to food hygiene, the latter seeing legislation appear in the 1870s in England to combat such things as the adulteration of food (Hardy 2001). Prior to this legislation red lead was added to cheese and mustard, and chalk to milk and flour with no legislative barriers (Halliday 2007). However, the cost of staple foods fell in the late 1800s as a result of cheap food sources from the colonies as well as Europe and the U.S. (ibid.). Halliday argues that the free-trade policies of the time had a positive effect here on the urban population, but a negative impact on British farmers.

Rickets was another major public health problem in the 1800s, a condition associated with poor nutrition and a lack of exposure to sunlight due to city smog. John Snow found children from all social classes suffering from rickets (Hardy 2001), and in 1884 every child examined at a Glasgow hospital had this condition (Halliday 2007). So although the wealthy could be protected from some conditions they were not protected from them all.[2]

In the nineteenth century the metaphor of 'laws' of public health became increasingly prominent, where disease and premature death were conceptualized as a just punishment for defying sanitary laws (Wood 2005). For some, diseases of poverty were seen as the result of economic laws, for which there was no remedy – a theory that was appealing to laissez-faire governments (Halliday 2007).

Laissez-faire attitudes were not the only ones at play in the nineteenth century. As noted in the introduction, Rudolf Virchow prescribed democracy and education as a cure for impoverishment (Halliday 2007). Links between public health and social justice were also evident in England, although they had less purchase on the rationale underpinning public health. For example, in the founding document of the 'Health of Towns Association', established in 1844, it stated that its goal was: 'To substitute health for disease, cleanliness for filth, order for disorder, economy for waste, prevention for palliation, justice for charity, enlightened self-interest for ignorant selfishness, and to bring to the poorest and meanest air, water and light' (cited ibid.: 25).

The 1848 Public Health Act in England and Wales put in place medical officers of health in urban centres, and in 1875 local government sanitary enforcement powers were made explicit (Hardy 2001). There was a shift at local government level from 'rate-payer-protective parsimony' to 'civic pride and civic competition' (ibid.: 31) around such issues as clean air, clean water and better working conditions.

In order to undertake public health works, such as the development of sewerage systems, coordination between local authorities in cities was required, and this fostered government centralization (Halliday 2007). But public health could not be sold to the public on the grounds of morality or public good alone, as anything requiring a tax on the population was negatively received. A view that investment in public health would save money was an argument proffered to gain assent to public health works (ibid.). For example, Chadwick, in the fourth annual report of the poor law commissioners, published in 1838, argued that epidemics meant charges were made on the poor rates. That is, diseases caused expenditure (ibid.). As such, a utilitarian argument based on economic efficiency was being advanced. In 1842 Chadwick's famous *Report on the Sanitary Conditions of the Labouring Population of Great Britain* was published. Here the costs of disease that led to 'the creation of widows, orphans, and those rendered incapable of work by diseases' were outlined (ibid.: 131). Immorality that arose from poor living conditions was also considered. Chadwick argued that insanitary conditions could turn 'the most cleanly and orderly female' into a 'gin-swilling drab' (cited ibid.: 191). City air pollution coupled with poverty would also lead to moral decline (Luckin 2002). Causation could be seen to go in the other direction as well, with immorality bringing on diseases such as cholera (Gilbert 2002). Over-indulgence in alcohol was believed to lead people to live in slum conditions which in turn were places of disease. Such beliefs meant that attention could focus on getting people to help themselves and become more disciplined, as opposed to providing them with financial assistance to obtain better housing.

The term 'sanitary' was first used in Chadwick's Report and as a concept it set new standards for healthy environments (Wood 2005). But sanitary environmental conditions to promote health also promoted morality – along the lines of the relationship between cleanliness and godliness (ibid.). For Chadwick the urban sources of physical depravity were also the source of moral depravity and crime (ibid.). However, the establishment position in the 1800s neglected the association between ill-health and poverty (Hardy 2001). The interwar years and the Depression led to some revision of this association, where the hardest hit U.K. areas in terms of economic depression had rising mortality levels (ibid.). The impact of poverty on health was further reinforced with the Second World War – where the effect of a more equal distribution of food through rationing measures led to a rising level of health amongst the poor (ibid.).

In noting the unsanitary conditions of the working class, Chadwick reported that there were two hundred thousand cesspools in London (Halliday 2007). Human waste was normally deposited in cesspools found in basements, and in London it was forbidden to dispose of such waste in rivers or sewers (ibid.). Cesspools were emptied at night by 'night soil men' who sold the waste on to farmers for fertiliser. Problems with cesspools were exacerbated by the introduction of water closets. In 1778 the valve water closet latrine was invented (Smith 2007). In Britain the Indian champu (shampoo) was introduced in the early eighteenth century through British Colonial India, as well as the shower bath (ibid.). Such developments and an increasing focus on cleanliness meant that larger volumes of flushed water filled up the cesspools much faster and made the contents much harder to transport, and much harder to sell to farmers as fertiliser (Halliday 2007).

To relieve households of overflowing cesspools Chadwick advocated the flushing of cesspools into the Thames. With this policy enacted, human waste with its waterborne infectious agents would return on the river tide to pollute the water supply – including the famous Broad Street pump (Halliday 2007). By 1850 nearly all human waste was disposed into common sewers. This in turn led to the 'great stink' of 1858 when the smell from the Thames was so vile that, given the understanding that disease was the product of miasma, it led to alarm over the health of parliamentarians who were subjected to it (ibid.). This hastened the introduction of sewerage systems to protect the water supply of Londoners and the collection of sewage sludge which was dumped in the North Sea (ibid.).

The 1848 Public Health Act in England and Wales permitted local authorities to take over water companies (Halliday 2007). Although this occurred infrequently in the initial decades after the act – it did signal a shift in thinking to public responsibility for such essential supplies, and by 1880 about half of the local authorities were running their own waterworks (ibid.). Public bath houses were also established in the mid-1800s – with some cities and charitable organizations establishing bath houses for the working classes (ibid.). Bath houses provoked unease in some sectors of Victorian England as they could turn into sites of debauchery, highlighting the tension between public and private spheres and morality in nineteenth-century public health discourse. Indeed, much of the push for public health was prompted by an interest in the moral well-being of the working class.

Gilbert argues that public health or public medicine that resulted from the sanitary movement 'initially meant state-supported health interventions, practised on behalf of a public formed of individual private citizens in whose service the state laboured and to whom it was accountable' (Gilbert 2002: 43). Private citizenship, in the 1800s, was not applied to everyone and therefore the state did not serve all. Citizenship was conceived as participation in the public sphere through the franchise, or voting rights, as well as participation in national culture through consumption. The 1832 Reform Act extended the voting franchise to householders who earned over ten pounds per annum, effectively excluding most workers (Host 1998). The 'lower working classes' were then not fully citizens as they did not have the minimal economic requirements to vote. It was not until the reform acts of 1867 and 1884 that the suffrage was extended to every adult male household member. Suffrage for women was not fully achieved until 1928. This lower class were disturbing as they did not practise bourgeois forms of domesticity. Work could take place in domestic spaces; and sleeping arrangements could mean sleeping with non-family members or with those of the opposite sex.

In rapidly urbanized spaces where traders and manufacturers might operate in residential areas, epidemiologists were enrolled to identify new threats to health. Nuisance inspectors became 'enforcers of bourgeois standards of the Victorian suburb quite as much as assailants of epidemic diseases' (Hamlin 2002: 198). In order to achieve this, 'nuisances' were required to be medicalized, thus providing public authorities with the legitimacy for interventions that could impinge upon trade or individual liberty (ibid.). From the 1830s, middle-class families were instructed on the subject of personal hygiene (Smith 2007: 277), which included stipulations to consume less food, be lean, and both mentally and physically fit. Improved standards of living had raised anxieties about corpulence or obesity. William James labelled the reformist nature of these anxieties the religion of 'healthy-mindedness' (ibid.). Trepidation about private health practices, particularly in relation to the rearing of children, led to the appointment of women health inspectors in the 1890s (Hardy 2001). There was increasing apprehension about the 'physical decrepitude of the average Londoner' (ibid.: 39). Home visits were then an intervention so that privacy and modesty could be learnt and bourgeois values inculcated (Gilbert 2002).

War and Health

As the nineteenth century progressed, Liberal arguments against public health steadily fell out of favour and public health became 'the most powerful justification for urban public action' (Hamlin 2002). Another impetus for public health interventions related to the fighting capacity of the nation-state.

During the nineteenth century Britain found itself in the midst of 'new imperialism'. The unification of Italy and Germany, and the resulting nationalistic sentiments, brought about an era of rapid and highly competitive colonialism. Since the American War of Independence, Britain had practised and encouraged trade with its many colonies and trading countries. Its superior navy and ability to raise vast capital in times of war provided sufficient protection from competing imperial powers. In this new era, competing states, particularly unified Germany which had become something of an industrial powerhouse, were aggressively seizing foreign territories with the intention of severely restricting trade (James 1994). British authorities became very nervous about the wealth of its empire, and responded with moves to formally secure many of the regions that, up until that time, had been ruled unofficially. If the empire was to remain strong and retain its wealth, it needed a fit and healthy population.

However, military screening revealed that this was lacking. A high rate of rejection of potential recruits for military service for the Boer War at the end of the nineteenth century clearly signalled a crisis in the physical degeneration of the British people (Hardy 2001). Throughout much of the Western world, worry about the health of the population became particularly salient during times of war. In 1928 a professor of education in the U.S. wrote: 'The Selective Service Draft for the World War showed that between thirty and forty per cent of the young men of the nation between twenty-one and thirty-one years of age were unfit for the duties of the army. They were, by that failure, also unfit for citizenship' (Feiring Williams 1928: 4).

This is a powerful statement linking health status to citizenship. Public health success in reducing death rates from infectious diseases was seen as one of the culprits of this situation – allowing the weak to survive and reproduce. Provision of services to women and children became more of a focus for local authorities during the First World War, as children, 'were, after all, the future source of cannon fodder' (Hardy 2001: 55).

At the end of the First World War it was argued that public health measures in England, particularly the provision of adequate housing, were an entitlement for those who had fought for King and Country. Under the phrase 'Homes Fit for Heroes', government policy changed to provide improved housing conditions for returning soldiers. Walter Long, a president of the Local Government Board in England stated 'to let them [the soldiers] come home from horrible, water-logged trenches to something little better than a pig-sty here would, indeed, be criminal ... A negation of all we have said during the war' (cited in Hardy 2001: 89).

Public health concerns were closely associated with military and economic concerns in nineteenth-century Paris. Efforts to create a healthier city and deal with cesspools and the droppings of thirty-seven thousand horses, which promoted pestilence and disease, also cleared out districts that were known for revolutionary resistance (Scott 1998). In the twenty-five years prior to 1851, barricades had gone up nine times in Paris, and those districts where revolutionary ferment was at its most fervent were the subject of city planning measures that expelled the occupants (ibid.).

New Imperialism brought about a French fixation on national health. France had been humiliated by its defeat in the Franco-Prussian war. Subsequently, there was a movement within France to revive the masses, so that a strong, competitive and prosperous nation would emerge. In order to regenerate the French people, an overhaul of the cities was needed, which could not go on being 'death chambers and cesspools' (Latour 1994: 19). Clean and dry rebuilt cities, with drains and fountains, schools, parks, gymnasiums and day nurseries were required (ibid.). As one advocate put it, an upheaval of the cities would harmonize 'national health' with 'national prosperity' and 'morality' (Stokes cited ibid.: 19). A hygienist movement took up the cause of Louis Pasteur and his disciples who were advocating the germ theory of disease and the establishment of corresponding public health measures aimed at the social regeneration of the nation. The 1902 Public Health Law was passed, enabling state authorities to act in the name of public health. Smallpox vaccination was made compulsory, doctors were legally required to notify officials of outbreaks of contagious diseases, and mayors were invested with the authority to ensure the supply of safe drinking water (Nord 1994).

American Exceptionalism

In contrast, the U.S.A.'s non-interventionism in European affairs meant that it was largely immune to the forces of competitive nationalism characteristic of late-nineteenth-century Europe. Poverty and ill-health were widespread, particularly in the large urban centres. Public health in the U.S. gained impetus from President Herbert Hoover's late-1920s national programme to abolish poverty. Hoover's aim was to establish what he called the 'Great Society of America'. This required reducing poverty, which could only be achieved, he argued, by applying scientific research to social problems (Bloom 2002: 5).

Hoover sought to ameliorate a 'shocking lack of data on which to base policies for coping with social problems' by forming what came to be known as the President's Committee on Social Trends (Bloom 2002: 58–59). The Committee, composed of many well-known scientists and social scientists of the time, aimed to develop the tools and methods necessary for large-scale population surveys. Meetings were held with local, state and federal officials as well as the very powerful philanthropists. Its major achievement was the production of a huge two-volume report comprising data on health statistics collected from both state and federal agencies, and importantly, a series of recommendations for tackling disease. These included better organization of health services by establishing effective coordination between government and health agencies, and improving professional training by teaching the prevention of disease. The report represented the first formulation of a national health programme. By ordering the coordination of health institutes and professionals with state and federal agencies it facilitated the expansion of the role of the government into health care, focusing heavily on disease prevention.

In the U.S., early public health, and indeed medicine as a whole, was closely tied to industrial capitalism. The great philanthropists, such as Carnegie and Rockefeller, donated millions of dollars to health and medicine via the establishment of trusts. Rockefeller, in particular, was a believer in the efficiency movement, where money was carefully directed towards areas that were deemed to be capable of generating some sort of social return, and was not consequently squandered on 'unwise' educational projects. Public health was seen as a means of establishing a strong, working population, necessary for powering the corporate and industrial U.S.A. that was emerging (Brown 1994). As an economist and the director of one of Rockefeller's trusts put it: 'Where mass diseases are brought under control, productivity tends to increase – through increasing the percentage of adult workers as a proportion of the total population [and] through augmenting their strength and ambition to work' (May cited ibid.: 116).

The type of medicine and public health that was deemed to be an efficient use of funds tended to focus on the individualistic, biological causes of disease. Approaches that embraced the work of Pasteur and Robert Koch and perpetuated the germ theory of disease often acquired funding. In contrast, those approaches that explained disease as the consequence of social and economic conditions, particularly those brought about by the industrial transformation, were ignored (Brown 1994). This led some commentators, such as Richard Brown, to claim that by funding medicine and health care, the rising industrialists were able to legitimize and disseminate their vision of the world. Contemporary medicine in the U.S. is still tainted with this focus on individualistic, biological causes of disease (ibid.).

Stocktaking

For many countries, military screening provided a means to do a stock check of the bodies of a large section of the population. Governments soon realized just how vital this sort of information was, and Hoover's establishment of the President's Committee on Social Trends can be seen as an example of such centralized surveillance. The British Liberal Government had also seen the worth in stocktaking its population. In 1905 it introduced legislation that set the foundations of public health surveillance in the U.K. This legislation established a system of medical inspection of schoolchildren, and required notification of births that enabled health visitors to supervise the first days of a child's life (Hardy 2001). The consequence of this fascination with the health of the population was that all bodies became potentially pathogenic, not just the diseased, bed-ridden body.

The rise of the modern hospital also had implications for public health. In the early twentieth century, hospitals became the main centres for medical treatment, and contained specialized departments for dealing with different types of illness. While in the nineteenth century health practitioners often worked alone in small communities, in the hospital health professionals were often required to work in conjunction with one another (Berg and Harterink 2004). Medical records became a vital part of medical practice. It soon became common procedure for every patient to have their own record, to which nurses and doctors would add progress notes, standardized forms and graphs containing test results, as well as a detailed description of the patient's affliction (ibid.). The establishment of a widespread system of records provided health professionals with a resource that revealed the frequency and history of ailments among large groups, and this made possible a general knowledge of population health (ibid.).

This enabled a whole new set of medical investigations that have subsequently played a vital role in the development of public health, such as statistical epidemiology in the 1950s. Ground-breaking findings like the link between lung cancer and smoking were made possible. Prior to such methodological developments as the prospective cohort study the cause of the increase in lung cancer rates was disputed. Atmospheric pollution was thought to be a cause (Hardy 2001). But by the 1950s epidemiological studies finding that the major cause of lung cancer was smoking were widely accepted in medical circles. Despite this, resistance from state and commercial interests hindered public health interventions for some time (see chapter 2 for further discussion of tobacco control). It took until 1965 before the U.K. banned smoking advertising on television, yet the death rate from the lung cancer epidemic continued to rise. Government resistance to strong enforcement measures against tobacco consumption have been linked to the substantial tax take from cigarette consumption – 4 billion pounds annually in the U.K. in the 1980s (Hardy 2001). Powerful economic interests were also able to stave off legislation limiting commercial activities in other areas where the evidence was less compelling than that relating to tobacco – such as the toxicity of food additives, pesticides, saturated fat consumption in food, and alcohol intake (ibid.).

Colonial Public Health and Eugenics

Approaches to public health in Britain's colonies were originally influenced by developments in the 'mother country', however, due to the impact of colonization there was a subsequent massive decline in the numbers of indigenous peoples in Canada, U.S.A., Australia, New Zealand and elsewhere. Indigenous peoples were often portrayed as dying races. The loss of land to settlers meant poverty, malnutrition and overcrowding for many, and a greater susceptibility to disease and population collapse (Reid 1999). The view that indigenous people would naturally die out meant that little was done to deal with their health problems before the early 1900s. At other times the settlements of indigenous populations, such as Māori pa in New Zealand, were portrayed as a threat to the whole country as they were seen as 'hotbeds' of disease (Bryder 1982). The theory of Social Darwinism was a prominent feature in directing public health efforts away from indigenous populations (Barta 2005). Social Darwinism fostered a view that the colonies were settled by robust immigrants, whilst the less robust indigenes suffered from ill health (Lange 1999). Such views would give support to those who would not want to intervene to help indigenous populations during a time when their numbers were declining. The decline was seen as natural and as a result of the survival of the fittest race – the European colonizers.

During early colonial history, there were many areas that were rife with disease. Colonial cities, such as Christchurch in New Zealand, were often badly drained and suffered 'from the effects of years of soil pollution from house slops and human excrement' (Maclean 1964: 349). Like their home countries, public health measures in settler societies were not based on compassion for humanity, but were enacted so the country could prosper and win future wars (Bryder 1982). The main focus was on improving the racial stock and national efficiency. The enfeebled and weakened state of the general population threatened the racial superiority of the settlers.

A 'problem' identified in the early 1900s that required a remedy was the bad housekeeping of women. The influenza epidemic of 1918 that killed millions throughout the world was seen by some as an outcome of women not being able to look after their families properly (Bryder 1982). In response, domestic science classes were promoted in schools (ibid.). Home nursing instruction was carried out by nurses. The rationale behind such measures was that women would elevate the race as married mothers would be trained by nurses to ensure that the white race would be healthy and thrive.

With an increasing national and ethnic mix in settler-society urban centres, racism and public health ideas began to merge. During the influenza pandemic of 1918, a New Zealand newspaper in the city of Auckland accused 'Hindoo hawkers' of spreading the disease 'for they take their stock of fruit to their awful dens everyday, where they fester in darkness and vileness, and sell them to the citizens of Auckland the next day' (Bryder 1982). In the early 1900s fear was expressed that clearing slums may force people to rent rooms from 'Chinamen' (ibid.).

The association of population health with the strength of the nation became most extreme in various eugenics movements. Anxiety about the physical deterioration of the British population led to the foundation of the Eugenics Education Society in 1907 (Smith 2007). The apotheosis of these links between the state and public health could be seen in Nazi fascism, which valorized physical beauty and fitness along with eugenics, and initiated anti-smoking campaigns, hygienic public health and cancer screening (ibid.). The lack of focus in public health discourse on issues such as disabilities and rare or inherited disorders (Forman 2008) may be evidence of a continuing trace of Social Darwinism.

Human Action and Disease

The history of public health, then, is not simply the adoption and application of scientific and medical principles by a benevolent government. This would be strikingly obvious if there was not a tendency to view science, technology and medicine as simple instruments that can be utilized to solve the problems of the day; as a set of tools that human actors can use to ameliorate various ills. Instead, it is more appropriate to see science, technology and medicine as playing a much more transformative and therefore inherently political role. As new technologies are adopted, they bring about novel social and material relations. These present previously unforeseen opportunities for action, and a host of new problems which are quite different to those of previous eras. With this sort of transformation, disease patterns change, and so do the tactics employed to deal with them.

For example, with the globalization of the world economy and the increasing traffic between nations, diseases can be spread more swiftly. The 'Black Death' first arrived in Europe in 1347, killing about a third of the entire population (Halliday 2007). Future visitations were less destructive, but continued with San Francisco and Sydney dealing with outbreaks as late as the 1900s. More recently, the used tyre trade has provided a means of exporting mosquitoes around the globe, which are capable of spreading a range of diseases including malaria and Ross River virus (Eberhart-Phillips 1999).

The impact of human activity leading to global warming is also likely to change disease patterns. Warming may encourage the spread of mosquitoes into areas where they have not previously been able to survive. This possibility is likely to be particularly problematic as malaria becomes increasingly resistant to the drugs used to fight the disease (Eberhart-Phillips 1999).

The threat of infection can also be influenced by government policy. For example, changes to housing policy during the 1990s in New Zealand, where the poor were forced to pay market rents for state housing, led to an increase in the number of two-family households. This overcrowding coincided with an escalation in the incidence of infectious diseases, including tuberculosis and meningococcal disease (Eberhart-Phillips 1999). Other infectious diseases can spread due to human behaviour, for instance, Hepatitis C transmitted by needle-sharing drug users (ibid.).

Concern about these infectious diseases is exacerbated by the view that we may be moving into a 'post-antibiotic' era. Powerfully illustrating how the adoption of technology has transformed the social and biological milieu, infectious agents have developed resistance to antibiotics. The most well known is dubbed the 'superbug' – *methicillin resistant staphylococcus aureus* (MRSA). Hospitals are the most likely places to encounter the superbug strain (Eberhart-Phillips 1999). It has been argued that there are many reasons for the development of antibiotic resistance. Penicillin was first made available to the British public in 1945, but penicillin-resistant strains of bacteria had already been identified by then, and the first signs of resistance to streptomycin were apparent in 1946 (Hardy 2001). Resistant strains have become increasingly common due the selective pressures brought about by the extensive use of antibiotics. It has been argued that this is the result of demanding patients insisting on inappropriate prescriptions, and profligate use of antibiotics to enhance growth in farm animals (Eberhart-Phillips

1999). It has been reported that the developing resistance of infectious agents may be hastened by the use of antibacterial products in household goods found in some cleaners, soaps and detergents (ibid.). In 2007 it was stated in the *Scientific American* that the increasing use of antibacterial soaps and other antibacterial products in households, instead of the traditional use of soap and hot water to remove dirt, may be creating conditions that promote resistant bacteria (Ballantyne 2007).

Much of public health is based on the notion that we can control nature for our benefit. However, there are occasions where unexpected outcomes of efforts to control nature have occurred. The eradication of smallpox allowed sustained outbreaks of an equally deadly monkeypox in parts of Central and West Africa. Prior to the eradication of smallpox the disease would confer immunity to monkeypox (Eberhart-Phillips 1999).

In many countries there has been unease about some vaccines used, and with an ever-increasing vaccine schedule these concerns are not likely to fade away. The polio vaccine is an 'attenuated' virus, which can on occasion become virulent causing polio. This has had the consequence that in some countries the only polio cases are caused by the vaccine. In Nigeria it was reported in 2007 that a polio vaccination programme had resulted in sixty-nine children being paralysed with polio (Cheng 2007). A question is then raised over when, if ever, it is appropriate for health authorities to cease using particular vaccines. This is particularly difficult as in some countries the wild virus is still a problem. In times of social and political breakdown, such as has occurred in some ex-Soviet Union states and in Albania, the wild polio virus has reappeared (Eberhart-Phillips 1999). In the case of Nigeria, due to concerns that the polio vaccination was an American plot to sterilize Muslims, the vaccination campaigns were cancelled in 2003. This led to an increase in the number of cases of polio not only in Nigeria, but also in surrounding countries (Cheng 2007). The findings, six years later, that the polio vaccine itself can also cause polio, as noted above, provides a particular hurdle for health authorities in their efforts to eradicate polio.

Public Health Policy

We live in very different circumstances from those that were at play during the early development of modern public health. Within public health practice the reassertion of the health inequalities agenda has not displaced the lifestyle agenda (Mooney 2008). Models of the social determinants of disease incorporate socio-economic, cultural and environmental conditions acting as a distal influence on health, impinging upon the more proximal influences on health that could include social and community networks that in turn influence individual lifestyle factors (Dahlgren and Whitehead 1991).

Several prominent concerns characterize the application and provision of contemporary public health. Firstly, there is ongoing debate about whether individual 'lifestyle', social determinants, or the specific biological disease should be the focus of public health measures. Secondly, with the prevalence of neo-liberalism and the corresponding shift of activities from the public to the private realm, there is considerable concern about how much power should be exercised by a government over individual citizens.

There has been renewed interest in public health in recent years, brought about mainly by the epidemic of chronic disease (Hunter 2007b). In developed countries, this began in the 1970s, where public health was revitalized as a result of rising health care costs and worry about the impact of modern lifestyles and 'diseases of comfort' (ibid.: 9). The publication in 1974 of the Lalonde Report in Canada heralded the dawn of 'new public health' (ibid.). Lalonde was the Canadian Health Minister at the time and the report provided a critique of reliance on the biomedical model of health care. The report had an 'upstream' focus calling for improvements in the environment and moderating lifestyles. It has been a rallying call in health promotion, but it failed to bring about any fundamental change in health policy which has continued to focus on health services (ibid.). In 1978 the WHO declared its aim of health for all by the year 2000 (Hardy 2001). The WHO focus was not on the provision of medical services but on the social determinants of health such as housing and education to improve health (discussed further in chapter 2) (ibid.).[3]

In 1980 the *Black Report* was published in Britain, demonstrating class-related disparities in health (Hardy 2001). The authors explain these disparities as arising from poverty and material deprivation, the solution to which required a radical redistribution of resources (ibid.). But the identification of redistribution of material resources as a public health intervention has had little purchase. For example, England's first health strategy – *Health of the Nation* – of 1992 advocated a disease-focused approach rather than one that focuses on social determinants of health, like the social inequalities in a society. By 1997 the presence of a Labour government in England made it acceptable to talk about the social determinants of health with a number of policies introduced to tackle social deprivation and poor health, such as 'Sure Start', neighbourhood renewal strategies and a minimum wage (Hunter 2007b). More recently, in the U.S.A. the Institute of Medicine asserted that 'health is a primary public good because many aspects of human potential such as employment, social relationships and political participation are contingent on it' (cited ibid.: 14) and that collective action was required, not individual responsibility.

However, the relation between public health and utilitarian principles still plays out. In the U.K., the 2002 report *Tackling Health Inequalities*, known as the Wanless Report, argued that public health action could increase productivity in the working population – so that good health made good economic sense (Hunter 2007a). This coincided with research highlighting contemporary public health scares around the impact of obesity, alcohol and sexually transmitted diseases on population health (ibid.). A political climate of giving patients and the public more choice goes against the grain of government-led public health interventions, and the 2004 White Paper *Choosing Health: Making Healthier Choices Easier* indicates in its very title that the emphasis was on facilitating people to make better choices rather than imposing legislation that would restrict behaviours – such as smoking bans (ibid.). Social marketing principles were preferred, that emphasized personal achievement (ibid.). The disinclination to centralize control in the state is seen in the reluctance of England to ban smoking in public places. Hunter argues that the ban in England only occurred after bans were in place in Scotland, Wales and Northern Ireland, and argues that Scotland has taken a lead in public health through the linking of public health agendas to social justice and environmental sustainability (Hunter 2007b).

What we see in these events is the shifting grounds of public health policy, which has gone through a rapid series of changes pivoting around a number of dichotomies: individual lifestyle and social determinants; personal responsibility and government regulation; increasing productivity and enhancing social justice.

Discussion

Morality, manners, morbidity and mortality were interwoven with the processes of urbanization and colonization of the nineteenth century, at the time that the founding myths of modern public health were established. Public health and epidemiology is a discipline replete with heroes: John Snow the founding hero, and additionally William Farr who developed statistical approaches to the study of population health, and Joseph Goldberger who discovered the cause of pellagra and related this to conditions of poverty and malnutrition in the southern states of the U.S.A. (Susser 1998).

The heroic vision of the public health researcher identifying causes of epidemics or railing against social injustice belies the complexity of public health. Early legislative developments and state actions in relation to public health alert us to a number of issues. We can see how social attitudes in relation to race, gender and class influence the sort of policies that are developed. We can see how issues of public health interweave with state power. The potential conflict between individual freedom and a well-intentioned state in relation to public health continues to be a point of contention today (Feingold 1998).

The relationship between science and public health is variable. Public health interventions that have a positive health impact can be based on 'false' understandings of the biological and social world. The 'paradigmatic' case in point might be that of sanitary reform in the nineteenth century, with all its positive outcomes for population health, being based on the miasmatic theory of causation (Susser 1998). Alternatively, a dogmatic adherence to particular beliefs can have negative outcomes. The discovery by Ignaz Semmelweis that washing hands could reduce the high fatality rates from puerperal fever in obstetric hospitals was rejected by his colleagues, as it did not fit with the accepted theory of miasmata in the air as the cause of infectious diseases (Porter 2006a). Public health can 'work' when the explanations for cause and effect are 'wrong', and equally adherence to 'orthodox' explanations can hinder public health. Explanations tying changes in life expectancy and declines in mortality to public health interventions can also be found wanting. Similarly the relationship between technological developments and public health are not linear. An illustrative example is the expansion in the use of water closets facilitating the demise of cesspools in basements, but carrying diseases into waterways with devastating consequences.

Public health, and its core discipline of epidemiology, has evolved through many stages. As public health came into being, that is, where the prevention and control of population health started to make a major impact during a time of rapid industrialization, the miasmatic theory of causation dominated. This was then superseded by the germ theory. The germ theory has not been displaced, but with the advent of the epidemiological transition and with chronic diseases becoming a more pressing concern than infectious diseases, it has been supplemented with risk factor epidemiology (Susser 1998). The evolution of public health continues, with molecular epidemiology as an example at one extreme, and global and international efforts to deal with broad social forces at the other (ibid.).

Sturdy argues that in the modern period the bourgeoisie not only used philanthropic institutions to domesticate the working class, but also appropriated local government institutions for that purpose (Sturdy 2002b). An argument made throughout this book is that public health can appropriate any means possible to facilitate its agenda to improve the health of the population. As such this can bring public health into conflict with the bourgeoisie and with capital, but also, at times, with the state where it has a laissez-faire agenda, and with the public it paternalistically seeks to save through forms of social engineering and the constraints it attempts to impose on the pursuit of, what many discursively articulate as, life's pleasures.

Considering public health and its development through the lens of a Durkheimian perspective provides some insights into the relationship that public health has with the state and the individual. Public health promotes certain kinds of restraint and as such is an important actor in contemporary society where the restraints of traditional forms of authority, such as religion, have been loosened. But in addition public health is in conflict with laissez-faire economics and so acts as a restraint to the free market, promoting the regulation of products and services that may work against the health of the public. The next chapter further explores the restraining aspects of public health in relation to trade, the global economy and social justice.

Notes

1. Interestingly, while Hygieia can be seen as the goddess of public health, her sister, Panacea, can perhaps be seen as the goddess equivalent of clinical medicine.

2. In chapter 5, Ulrich Beck's discussion of the Risk Society is introduced. Beck argued that one distinction between risk in contemporary society (such as from nuclear radiation or pesticide use) and risk in other societies is that it now affects all social classes. Previously risk was class specific, with the poor and the working classes exposed to more hazardous surroundings. The case of rickets is one example where this distinction does not hold in urban societies.
3. In 1907 the European office International D'Hygiene Publique was established that later became the League of Nations Health Organization Committee. This was replaced by the World Health Organization in 1948 (Smith 2007).

CHAPTER 2
The Politics of Public Health

Introduction

'Social injustice is killing people on a grand scale' (CSDH 2008) – so states the World Health Organization's Committee on the Social Determinants of Health. This chapter explores social justice in relation to representations of population health, knowledge production, commerce, the state, and international agencies. Public health activities can act to control populations or advocate for change at the state and international level. This is not without its contradictions and paradoxes. Public health can be used as a means of promoting social good, or as a means of opening up markets to commercial enterprise. Public health can resist the efforts of multinational companies to enrol populations in consumption behaviours that are likely to be harmful to health, and as such, to reinforce the rights of nationals and nation-states. But public health can also attempt to undermine the vagaries of national politics through external interventions and by advocating for international conventions.

Public health, in its goals and organizational forms, can cut across many jurisdictions. This can and has set up a number of tensions. There is a potential conflict between international health efforts to intervene to improve health and nation-states. The latter may assert their national sovereignty and resist public health efforts to expose the negative health impacts of government policy on populations. The capacity of epidemiology to graphically represent patterns of morbidity and mortality across time, social classes, ethnicity and a host of other variables can forcefully highlight the levels of social injustice within a nation-state and between nation-states.

Whereas nation-states can become limited and constrained by the imposition of neo-liberal programmes, public health can provide a source of resistance to these constraints. Public health advocates have been highly critical of international organizations whose impact has, arguably, increased social and therefore health inequalities. Policies of structural adjustment as advocated by the World Bank and the International Monetary Fund (IMF) have been accused of facilitating the devastating consequences of the AIDS epidemic in parts of Africa.[1] The opening up of Zambia to textile imports led to the demise of state-run clothing manufacturers. The privatization of state industries led to profits moving offshore to the foreign-owned firms rather than cross-subsidizing health, education and other social services. The political causes of economic decline facilitated the trading of sexual services for money as a means of survival, linking the pathological cause of the diseases to the political one (Labonté 2008). Critiques of this nature can be applied throughout the developing world. Public health advocates critique international organizations fostering a health-deteriorating neo-liberal structural adjustment agenda.

Public health is, then, a potential buffer against rampant capitalism as it adds to the argument for a need to regulate the economy and limit the extent of social inequality. These functions of public health align with the functions of Durkheim's cult of humanity. At the heart of the cult of humanity is a concern for social justice.

Representations and the Politics of Public Health

Social epidemiology points to the social causes of illness and death, and has the potential to influence policy goals directed at ameliorating negative social impacts on health. Classically, the social causes of morbidity and mortality have included unequal distributions in income, education, housing, work and working conditions, and other social factors that lead to unequal social outcomes (CSDH 2008). The science of social epidemiology, then, leads to calls for social justice in the policy arena. To reduce health inequalities social inequalities must also be reduced. A seminal publication in this regard was the *Black Report* (1980) in the U.K., which, like more recent U.K. reports highlighting the link between social and health inequalities, was a source of political embarrassment for the government of the day (Shaw et al. 2005), although, as noted in chapter 1, it had little immediate impact upon policy. A social epidemiology report published by the New Zealand Ministry of Health titled *Decades of Disparity* pointed at neo-liberal restructuring as a cause of widening health gaps between different groups (Ajwani et al. 2003; Blakely et al. 2005). Public health in this context offers a critique of the excesses of unregulated capitalism, performing an important function in a society based on social differentiation and individualism.

Compelling imagery of social injustice can be presented at a national level showing differences in life expectancy by occupation or social class, gender and ethnicity. Data collected can be presented to show consistent differences in life expectancy by gender across all occupational classes, with women living up to six years longer than men in England and Wales (Scambler and Scambler 2007). This difference in life expectancy by gender is common in all developed countries (Sandiford 2009). In England and Wales professional men have an eight-year advantage in life expectancy over unskilled working men (Scambler and Scambler

2007). The identification of different health outcomes by class have been of long-term interest in public health, going back to the nineteenth century. Identifying differences in health outcome by ethnicity has been more a product of the twentieth century. The capacity to collect data on life expectancy, relate it to demographic characteristics, and represent differences in visual form provides a basis for debate about causes and interventions within nation-states, and a capacity to monitor social policies that increase or reduce these differences. Further, the notion of the social gradient developed by social epidemiologists has led to conceptual thinking that always places the individual within a collective context. The idea that everyone in the population is somewhere on the social gradient, and therefore that inequalities affect everyone in society (Kawachi et al. 1999), is a profound vision of collectivity and a persuasive call to social justice.

Graphic representations of differences in life expectancy by ethnicity provide similar possibilities for policy debates. Gaps in life expectancy between indigenous groups and settler groups change over time (Ajwani et al. 2003). For example, data showing a gap between the non-Māori (settlers and their descendents) and Māori (indigenous population) in New Zealand demonstrates variation over time in the gaps in life expectancy that speak to fundamental social change, like shifts of populations from rural to urban areas, the impact of economic restructuring and how it differentially impacts on indigenous and non-indigenous groups, and so on. Life expectancy data and other data have the potential to hold governments accountable for social policies that fail to narrow the 'ethnic' gap in health outcomes.

Data collected or used by social epidemiologists can convincingly illustrate social injustice at an international level. There is a massive 40-year-plus gap in life expectancy between the richest and poorest countries. A baby boy born in Swaziland can expect to reach the age of 36, whereas one born in Japan can expect to reach the age of 79 (World Health Organization 2006). The magnitude of the injustice at play can be demonstrated where even a relatively small redistribution of wealth internationally could have a dramatic impact on the life expectancy of the poor and almost no negative health consequences for the rich countries. For the richer countries it takes a very large increase in income to obtain even a small increase in life expectancy (Deaton 2007).

Data generated by epidemiological research are powerful stimuli to calls for social justice. The changes in life expectancy for the different population groups are not easily explained by individual lifestyle choice or changes in health service delivery, although all these may play some part at particular times or for particular conditions. Rather, these representations speak to structural, organizational and policy factors and the collective efforts of society that facilitate more or less just health outcomes.

The State and Public Health

Public health, social justice and the democratic state were closely linked long before the development of epidemiology. The 1792 declaration of the French National Assembly, that health was a right, provided the basis for population health endeavours in democratic societies (Porter 2008). At the same time, the Assembly declared work a right. Porter argues that the relationship between work and population health continued to play out during later centuries. Industrializing societies required a labour supply, and so public health measures to reduce mortality from infectious diseases became a political priority (ibid.). Later the increasing impact of caring for the chronically sick overrode prior concerns about infectious diseases in wealthier countries (ibid.).

Public health historians have taken different views on the role of the state in relation to public health. Early analyses linked particular state types to public health strategies in a linear fashion. Erwin Ackerknecht suggested that, in relation to public health, authoritarian governments favoured quarantine whereas liberal governments preferred sanitationist policies (Gross Solomon et al. 2008). Later historians argued for much more complicated relationships between public health and the state, where other forces would shape and influence the strategies used, including the social structures and institutional features of nation-states (ibid.).

Baldwin argues that different nation-states do take different approaches to public health concerns related to the particular ethos and the social, political and economic circumstances of the nation-state (Baldwin 2008). The U.S. response to the AIDS epidemic was to concentrate on biomedical interventions that focused on nature rather than social interventions with a target of behavioural change (ibid.). This was, argues Baldwin, an outcome of a heterogeneous U.S. nation-state that contains within it a diversity of moral and religious standards; thus there was greater delicacy in dealing with behaviour change, encouraging other approaches to the epidemic. A more extreme example of a different approach to public health concerns is the case of South Africa's response to the AIDS epidemic. South African president, Thabo Mbeki, supported the views of AIDS denialists who believed that AIDS was not caused by HIV but by other factors, such as malnutrition or the use of antiretroviral drugs used to treat AIDS. It has been estimated that 343,000 deaths could have been prevented between the years 1999 and 2007 if South Africa had conformed to an orthodox public health approach to AIDS instead of pursuing policies based on this denialist position (Natrass 2008). In this instance, the failure of orthodox public health to achieve alignment with the state had devastating consequences.

Historically, as the state secured increasing command over the health of the public particular groups were empowered. As the medical profession became regulated in the nineteenth and twentieth centuries the state increasingly conferred powers upon it. As we saw in chapter 1, the state or local government required the medical profession to oversee efforts to improve the public health – the establishment of medical officers of health being a salient example. Doctors were given the role of providing scientific legitimacy to a series of legislative policies, including disease prevention, the supervision of hospitals and the control of food and drug legislation.

States deploy public health in different ways to control populations. Public health sanitary reform in the nineteenth century led to a limitation of private property rights, and the heated controversy over smallpox vaccinations provided a classic contest between public and individual goods (Baldwin 2008). State attempts to control particular populations, through public health measures, can have unintended outcomes. The responses to the contagious diseases acts in the nineteenth century, which acts can be regarded as an attempt by the state to deploy public health measures as a means of controlling women, provided the foundations for the women's movement (ibid.). The position of the medical profession improved as the state made attempts to control the lives and activities of women. Contagious diseases acts were passed in the 1860s, which treated women suspected of prostitution as being morally corrupt and medically unclean (Howell 2000). Magistrates were given the power to imprison women suspected of being prostitutes and could force them to undergo medical treatment (Wilson 1992). Doctors gained powers to enforce the hospitalization of prostitutes diagnosed with venereal disease, and also the right to medically inspect women suspected of being prostitutes (Belgrave 1985). There was no equivalent legislation aimed at men who frequented prostitutes.

This highlights a particular relationship between the state and the medical profession where the moral campaigns of the state may increase the professional power of medicine. Not only do we have the issue of how the state should treat a sufferer of a contagious disease when the sufferer is both a disease vector and a citizen (Baldwin 2008), but also how moral campaigns and the control of certain sections of the population link to public health.

The relationship between the state and public health in Germany through the twentieth century demonstrates the extremes that can be taken in this relationship. In the German public health service after the First World War the concept of social hygiene was promoted by left-wing physicians to call for reforms to living conditions (Schleiermacher 2008). As such, public health concerns were policy concerns. By the 1930s state-controlled health departments had been established, but in this instance the health policy system was founded on the concept of racial hygiene (ibid.). The Nazi regime had successfully achieved a national health policy, but in a form very different from those promoting national policies under the Weimar Republic. The Nazis drew on public health rhetoric to provide scientific arguments for programmes of genocide (Baldwin 2008).

In the German Democratic Republic in the postwar period health policy was conceived as a concern for all state institutions (Schleiermacher 2008), a forerunner of the contemporary development of health impact assessments (discussed in chapter 7). Within this socialist orientation the focus of health intervention was to protect and replenish the workforce (Schleiermacher 2008).

The epidemiological transition shifts the focus of public health interventions both within and across nation-states. Concerns related to the impact of this epidemiological transition can be seen as far back as the 1920s, when statisticians working for insurance companies examined relationships between lifestyle and morbidity and mortality (Porter 2008). In 1922 the Milbank Memorial Fund, which is an endowed foundation established in 1905 to advise the public and private sector on health policy, shifted its focus from philanthropy to a social science approach to public health. It concentrated on collecting information, developing intervention strategies to improve health in terms of the conditions of life such as housing and nutrition, determining the costs of sickness, and developing strategies to disseminate knowledge that promoted healthy lifestyles (Weindling 2008). This led to the development of community and family studies supported by the fund – including the U.S. Public Health Service study in Hagerstown, Maryland, between 1921 and 1924. This study was based on the random selection of two thousand families participating in six-weekly interviews for up to three years, with surviving families being surveyed again twenty years later (Lawrence and Tibbitts 1951). These studies identified the impact of morbidity in communities, such as the prevalence of respiratory conditions that were not so well reflected in mortality statistics (Weindling 2008). With these findings, chronic illness could become as much of a concern to public health interventions as attempts to reduce mortality.

Concerns about this epidemiological transition led to the establishment of the famous Framingham study of heart disease. The Framingham study was initiated in 1947. At the time, epidemiological knowledge of heart disease was poor (Oppenheimer 2005). In developing their framework of research, the study popularized the concept of risk factor epidemiology, highlighting, for example, the role of diet in diseases (ibid.; Porter 2008).

At a similar time, British research highlighted the role of exercise in relation to heart disease. In 1952, Harvard University hosted a symposium on 'Overeating, overweight, and obesity' (Porter 2008). Porter argues that these developments signalled a shift in the core concerns of public health from structural explanations to lifestyle ones (ibid.). The concern for lifestyle was profoundly demonstrated when the link between tobacco consumption and lung cancer was established by Richard Doll and Austin Bradford Hill – also in the 1950s. Porter argues that the way of managing chronic illness was to emphasize 'individual prevention, raising health consciousness, and promoting self-health care' (ibid.: 48). But more than this, Porter argues that 'the analysis of the relationship between smoking and lung cancer gave epidemiology new credibility as the authoritative source of a bio-, psycho-, socio-, medical model of chronic disease. It became a critical heuristic device, and legitimated a new approach to disease prevention through controlling individual's lifestyles' (ibid.: 48).

The extent of the dominance of healthy lifestyle promotion can be seen in the U.S. where the Combined Health Information Database had, in just a 4-month period in 2004, published nineteen hundred items on healthy lifestyle promotion (Porter 2008). Issues of weight, alcohol and drug consumption are examples of where targeting individual behaviour occurs, and some of the problems this gives rise to in the clinical consultation will be discussed in chapter 4.

But there was clearly another radical tradition in public health. Public health can tend towards a conservative focus on influencing lifestyles through education or it can tend towards a more radical focus calling for popular democracy, human rights and redistribution policies. In 1952, at the Fifth World Health Assembly, C.E.A. Winslow, professor emeritus of public health at Yale University, stated that 'Public health, like governments, must be "'of all the people' and 'by all the people' as well as 'for all the people'"' (cited in Murard 2008: 141).

Much earlier, during the interwar years, public health interventions in rural areas of Europe and the Americas supported indigenous development (Murard 2008). Disease prevention was to occur through the targeting of 'downtrodden villagers' (ibid.: 142). Public health initiatives in Yugoslavia in the 1920s supported 'imaginative nationalisms' amongst villagers which, besides the establishment of health cooperatives, included cultural cooperatives that reinvented traditions and reanimated music societies (ibid.: 148). Included as a member of the League of Nations Health Committee in the interwar years was Andrija Štampar, a Yugoslav who argued that 'radical changes of an economic and social order were necessary' to improve the health of the rural populations (Zylberman 2008). Public health interventions were not simply about changing individual behaviour, but were community-oriented programmes that went beyond the specifics of public health sanitary and disease prevention strategies. Such approaches were taken up and applied in India and elsewhere. As such, Murard argues that 'social medicine increasingly nurtured the Third World aspirations that had become molded into an ideological hunger for nationhood' (Murard 2008: 154).

The radical nature of public health is encapsulated in that John Grant, a member of the International Health Board of the Rockefeller Foundation, could style himself as a medical Bolshevik (Murard 2008). He believed that 'public health was an integral part of socioeconomic progress' (Bu and Fee 2008). This contrasted with the Rockefeller Foundation's conventional conception of public health as narrowly focused technical interventions (Birn 1999). Grant's methods for training health workers in China served as a model for the barefoot doctor. One of Grant's public health concerns was to keep high technology medicine at bay. This position, taken up in radical form by one of his students, C.C. Chen in North China, led to the development of the training of village aides in ten days, in order to replace the need to support expensive physicians (Murard 2008). China introduced a barefoot doctor system in 1958, which was a system of rural health workers who undertook a range of activities, including anti-epidemic work. The training of barefoot doctors took substantially less time than the training of conventional doctors and could be part-time and on-the-job (Koplan et al. 1985).

Thus public health interventions could foster a process of deprofessionalizing medical practice. This yet again points to the different outcomes facilitated by the diverse relationships that public health has with the state and with, in this case, the profession of medicine. In the developed world public health concerns of the state bolstered the professionalizing strategies of medicine, but in China it threatened this professional status.

Murard argued from his studies of public health conferences in the interwar years that at that time public health was not a unitary entity (Murard 2008). At various stages public health interventions could be based on the promotion of nationalism, at others on internationalism. In relation to radical politics, public health could support indigenous populations and resist the imposition of expertise, including efforts that would deprofessionalize doctors, and it could equally put in efforts on the international stage to prevent war – as various public health agencies did prior to the Second World War (ibid.).

With great improvements in health outcomes throughout the last century, the health gap between the rich and poor has widened in some countries – like the U.K. (Evans 2007). In the U.K., two reports have often been cited for their role in highlighting inequalities in health outcomes by social class. The *Black Report* of 1980 reported on class gradients for almost all causes of death, and the *Acheson Report* of 1998 reported that the inequalities had further widened (ibid.). But in some countries inequalities are much smaller, as for example, in Sweden (ibid.). The argument made by public health researchers is that such differences are the result of forms of social organization, questioning the lifestyle approach to public health. Sweden has pursued policies of equality in the social and labour market spheres, and this reduction of inequality in these spheres also reduced inequalities in health outcomes (ibid.).

Such findings have led to a great deal of theorizing and research activity around the causal pathways that explain these health inequalities. How much can be explained by behavioural risk factors, how much by the psychological impact of inequality (the psycho-social hypothesis) and how much as a result of material poverty (Evans 2007)? Well-known and well-respected public health researchers, such as George Davey-Smith, have called for income redistribution policies to end poverty and end inequalities in health (ibid.). Such concerns about the impact of social policy on health outcomes draw public health advocates into the policy arena, where lobbying activities become an important feature in public health work (ibid.).

From a public health research perspective the current forms of legitimacy in clinical health research do not allow for strong statements to be made about the impact of policy on health outcomes. As Davey-Smith states, 'The Cochrane Library is unlikely ever to contain systematic reviews or trials of the effects of redistributive national fiscal policies, or on economic investment leading to reductions in unemployment, on health' (cited in Evans 2007: 164).[2]

Public health can have more radical and more conservative forms today. Lifestyle interventions and risk factor epidemiology can foster a focus on the individual, but explicit examples of a radical positioning of public health are readily found in journals like *Critical Public Health* and the *International Journal of Health Services*.

International Public Health

The contemporary international focus of public health is wide ranging. A strong emphasis is on disease surveillance and rapid alert and response systems, but it can also include such international agreements as the Montréal Protocol of 1986 banning Chlorofluorocarbons (CFCs) (Orme et al. 2007b).

It was not until after the First World War that international activity on public health took off (Gross Solomon et al. 2008). An Office International d'Hygiène Publique was established in Paris in 1907, but it did not really operate in an international way. Rather, it provided a forum for officials from different countries to come together (ibid.). International public health efforts could be met with suspicion by nation-state representatives. The League of Nations established a Health Organization (LNHO) in 1920. In 1922 a British member of the health committee of the LNHO expressed concern about the workings of such an institution, stating that 'the conception of a superepidemiologist at Geneva seems radically unsound' (cited in Gross Solomon et al. 2008: 11). The vision of a superepidemiologist promotes anxiety over state sovereignty and the autonomy of localized public health.

The British traditions of liberalism and national sovereignty were seen as being under threat from the League of Nations' Health Organization between the world wars – with the LNHO's social approach and focus on state responsibilities for the health of populations being a particular concern (Borowy 2008). U.S. agencies were not so reticent, with the Senate Committee on Education and Labour arguing that improved world health would increase U.S. markets (ibid.).

In efforts to eradicate malaria from Mediterranean countries in the interwar years, Lewis Wendell Hackett, an International Health Commissioner with the Rockefeller Foundation, wrote: 'Of course I believe in sanitation through evolution, education and prosperity … But with a backward people, I believe in a preliminary cleaning up through strict enforcement of sanitary code, whether the people thoroughly understand it or not! This is easier in a colony or under a mandate than in a democracy' (cited in Zylberman 2008: 283).

This technical solution to public health problems can be contrasted with the radical public health positions and other positions taken even within the Rockefeller Foundation. During the 1920s the Rockefeller Foundation attempted to develop public health strategies in such a way as to support self-sustaining democratic communities. This raised suspicions from conservatives that the preventive arm of public health in terms of improving sanitary conditions was in fact socialized medicine (Weindling 2008).

International health agencies, like national public health agencies, have variously focused on the technical aspects of disease control and eradication, and the social aspects of behaviour change, and environmental change (the environment here including the political). The constructivist school of international relations has pushed the view that health agencies primarily foster norms of 'cooperation and altruistic social improvement' (Gillespie 2008). In other words, an attempt is made to involve international public health in changing social norms but without meddling in national politics. But international public health efforts were used by the U.S. and its allies to establish and maintain politically sympathetic regimes after the Second World War (ibid.). This usually involved a technical approach – for example, major campaigns along the lines of a military organization to eradicate mosquitoes in Sardinia.

Governments were also wary of efforts by international agencies, such as the League of Nations, to measure health conditions in communities as this could expose issues of social deprivation (Weindling 2008). To expose such issues would not only cause embarrassment for a particular government but could foment rebellion and calls for social change and radical reform.

The social approach to public health was apparent in the founding documents of the WHO (Borowy 2008: 104). The Alma Ata conference of 1978 is regarded as a watershed in public health activities at an international level. It was at this international conference on Primary Health Care in the Soviet Union that WHO's very broad definition of health was adopted, with health conceived of as being a state of physical, mental and social well-being, not just the absence of disease and disability (World Health Organization Regional Office for Europe 1985). At this conference the goal was set for governments to attain a level of health for all by 2000 that would allow socially and economically productive lives.

The principles of equity underlying Alma Ata, with a focus on the social determinants of health including education, housing and food provision, were thought to be a mechanism to 'reduce the scope of politics' (Gross Solomon et al. 2008: 2). In other words, international public health efforts were situated as buffering nation-states against the vagaries of national politics – tempering the absolutist tendencies of the state.

Developments that have come under the rubric of globalization have challenged the traditional focus of public health on issues within national borders (Collin and Lee 2007). The concept of 'transborder health risk' encapsulates issues related to the challenge, that is, risks that transcend jurisdictional boundaries. These risks are posed by different vectors, and can include organisms that carry infections or corporate businesses that trade in lethal or disease-promoting products.

The AIDS epidemic provided for a reinvigoration of public health on the international arena by demonstrating the 'epidemiological interconnectedness of the world' (Baldwin 2008: 24). Baldwin argues that '[t]he developed world outsourced its unfulfilled sexual needs – both gay and straight – to the Third World, then harvested the epidemiological results'. In 2002 and 2003 severe acute respiratory syndrome (SARS) caused widespread panic around the globe as it spread out from China before it was contained and eliminated through old-fashioned public health quarantine measures (ibid.). Throughout much of the developed world there was a rapid decline in the rates of tuberculosis (TB) infection after the Second World War, but this decline plateaued in the 1980s. One of the main sources of TB in developed countries was migrants from high TB-incidence countries (Das et al. 2006).

Due to the porous borders of nation-states, public health systems cannot have a 'fortress' mentality of protecting the population within the border, but instead need to address issues from a global perspective (Collin and Lee 2007). Even relatively isolated countries, like New Zealand, failed in their containment strategies in relation to the so-called swine 'flu epidemic of 2009. The HN51 virus could not be stopped without halting all international travel.

Public health has also engaged with concerns about the possible exacerbation of inequalities as a result of the expansion of global markets. Currency speculators have been pointed to as a major threat to global public health (McClean 2007). The establishment of the World Trade Organization in 1995 put in place agreements that favoured the transnational corporations of richer nations (Labonté and Torgerson 2008). Its focus on removing barriers to trade and expanding private markets is seen as a threat to state efforts to combat health inequalities (McClean 2007).

One goal of trade liberalization is to expand private provision of services and open these services to foreign ownership – and these services include education and health (McClean 2007). WHO potentially stands in opposition to international moves that have the potential to exacerbate inequalities – but has been accused of being an impotent player in relation to trade liberalization (ibid.). The tension between trade and health is perhaps most pronounced in relation to tobacco.

The Politics of Tobacco Control

The link between cancer and environmental exposures has a long history. In 1775 Percival Pott claimed a causal link between soot exposure to chimney-sweeps and cancer of the scrotum (Lippman and Hawk 2009). But making such links is a controversial process. Public health is clearly not simply a matter of applying knowledge in a neutral way in order to enhance the health of people. Public health knowledge is produced within a particular social, political and cultural environment. When attempts are made to bring about changes for public health reasons, different groups in any society will support or reject those changes. The politics of public health is well illustrated with the example of tobacco control. Tobacco policy demonstrates the complex relations between knowledge production in public health and intervention strategies that span across the globe. Tobacco is an excellent example of how public health can come into conflict with the logic of capitalism.

In the U.S. it was noted that lung cancer deaths were steadily increasing from the early part of the twentieth century. In the 1930s there were fewer than three thousand deaths per year from lung cancer, but by 1962 this had grown to forty-one thousand (Pratt 2004). Two contending theories were proposed to explain the increase: atmospheric pollution as lung cancer was more prevalent in the cities, and smoking cigarettes. Richard Doll and Austin Bradford Hill initiated their prospective cohort study of British doctors in 1951 – and within five years a relationship between smoking and lung cancer, as well as between smoking and coronary heart disease, was identified (ibid.). In 1957 the Medical Research Council in Britain published a statement claiming a direct causal link between smoking and lung cancer.

But this was not universally accepted. Some scientists were unconvinced that the association proved causation, such as R.A. Fisher, who was regarded as one of the most eminent biological statisticians of his time (Pratt 2004). There were also discrepancies in the research, including a finding that those doctors who did not inhale were more likely to get cancer. Alternative hypotheses to the one that smoking caused cancer included one that proposed that there was a genetic predisposition to smoke and to having lung cancer (or confounding in epidemiological terms). Another hypothesis proposed that lung cancer causes smoking.

As a result of these disputes over the relationship between smoking and lung cancer a Surgeon General's Advisory Committee on Smoking and Health was established in the U.S.A. in 1964. For this committee, 10 scientists were selected from a possible 150. To get to the final selection, both health groups and tobacco groups vetoed scientists from the original 150, and any scientists who had a public position on the topic were excluded. Even after the vetoing process one scientist from Harvard University was later found to have undeclared funding connections to the tobacco industry. However, the report from the committee concluded that smoking was causally related to lung cancer. The report was regarded as an authoritative statement on the topic.

Andy Pratt argues that a hindsight view has presented Fisher and other dissenters to the growing consensus around the causal link between smoking and lung cancer as being misguided, incompetent and puppets of tobacco companies. However, dissent in science is normal and crucial (Pratt 2004). Robert Merton's scientific norm of organized scepticism suggests that dissent, or at least critical scrutiny, is a requisite norm of science (Merton 1973), and that there is no clear line to demarcate dissent from misguidance or deceit – hence the ongoing debates in relation to the anthropogenic nature of climate change.

But public health cannot wait for scientific certainty. As Austin Bradford Hill states: 'All scientific work is incomplete – whether it be observational or experimental. All scientific work is liable to be upset or modified by advancing knowledge. That does not confer upon us a freedom to ignore the knowledge we already have, or to postpone the action that it appears to demand at the time' (cited in Pratt 2004: 231).

However, even prior to the 'resolution' of the dispute over the causes of lung cancer there was a long history of fighting tobacco consumption. Anti-nicotine societies were formed in the late 1800s to lobby for the prohibition of tobacco (Thomson and Wilson 1997). This was primarily on moral grounds in that tobacco was thought to have a corrupting influence (Jacobson et al. 1997). In the U.S. fourteen states had banned the production, sale and advertising of cigarettes by the early twentieth century, however these were either not enforced or were repealed (ibid.).

It was not until the 1950s that reports linking smoking to lung cancer and other health problems were widely circulated in the medical profession. It was not until the 1960s that public awareness about the health impacts of tobacco consumption was raised. Prior to this the medical profession was not strongly opposed to smoking. Although heavy smoking was thought to be a possible concern because it might be an irritant, it was also thought to have positive effects in helping people to relax, providing pleasure and increasing sociability (Thomson and Wilson 1999). Housewives were even encouraged to have a cigarette as a way of relaxing from their work. Up until the 1960s at least one cigarette company still made claims on their packaging that smoking does not affect heart or lungs.

The relationships of governments to tobacco and the tobacco industry have varied over time. Governments have taxed tobacco in order to obtain revenue and also encouraged tobacco farmers by protecting them with tariffs and helping them with research (Thomson and Wilson 1999). From the 1960s more effort was made to curb smoking, including television and radio bans on cigarette advertising. In the late 1970s research implicated the effects of passive smoking, which supported calls for banning smoking in public places.

In the mid-1970s, adult male smoking rates in a number of developed countries – including the U.K., U.S. and Canada – ranged from 42 to 54 per cent, and female rates from 31 to 41 per cent (Pierce 1989). In 1996 it was estimated that there were five million deaths per year worldwide that were attributable to smoking (Scally 2007) and it has been estimated that by 2030 tobacco use will kill ten million people annually (Shaffer et al. 2005). Over half of all persistent-smokers' deaths are attributable to smoking (Lippman and Hawk 2009). Such deaths are avoidable, with smoking regarded as 'the most important cause of preventable illness and death and inequalities in health' (Amos 2007).

In the U.S., from the 1990s, tobacco industry tactics began to be uncovered. The influence of tobacco companies came under a lot more scrutiny, and there was a great deal of lobbying at local, national and international levels to control and reduce tobacco consumption (Amos 2007). In effect, this directed attention to the activities of the tobacco industry, and attempts to repress and limit smoking were no longer limited to simply discouraging smokers through education and taxation. Tobacco industry documents that had been kept secret now revealed that the industry knew for decades that nicotine was addictive and that smoking caused a variety of diseases. The documents also revealed that the tobacco industry had used the power at its disposal to prevent this information getting out into the public and into the courts (Glantz and Balbach 2000). In other words, tobacco companies were caught suppressing information about the dangers of their product (Watterson 1994). A Hollywood depiction of this can be seen in the film *The Insider*.

As noted, at an international level there is a tension between international covenants which seek to promote health and well-being and international trade agreements which prioritize the rights of corporations (Shaffer et al. 2005). International regional and bilateral trade agreements are intended to reduce barriers to trade. In 1995 the World Trade Organization (WTO) was established, and through this organization binding agreements have been placed on its 148 member nations that impose strict rules on government regulation. The WTO put in place agreements that favoured the transnational corporations of richer nations (Labonté and Torgerson 2008).

Earlier still, a General Agreement on Tariffs and Trade (GATT) came into effect in 1948 and has been used to promote tobacco products. The U.S.A. threatened trade sanctions against countries in Asia, claiming that policies to limit tobacco consumption such as high tariffs and taxes, and advertising restrictions, unfairly limited the market for U.S. tobacco companies (Shaffer et al. 2005). Philip Morris threatened to launch a trade dispute against Canada in 1994 when Canada intended to introduce plain packaging of cigarettes. Canada withdrew the legislation (ibid.).

Eighty-two per cent of the world's smokers are in low-to-middle-income countries (Collin and Lee 2007). Trade liberalization, under the threat of U.S. retaliatory trade sanctions, led to an increase in per capita tobacco consumption of 10 per cent in the previously closed markets of Japan, Taiwan, South Korea and Thailand between 1986 and 1991 (ibid.).

International public health agencies have, however, fought back. In 2003 the World Health Assembly endorsed the Framework Convention on Tobacco Control (FCTC). Collins and Lee argue that the FCTC is an exemplar of new forms of governance in response to globalization. This framework was the first attempt by WHO to use a legal strategy to improve population health and includes measures that clearly aim to restrict the trade in tobacco (McClean 2007). Features of this convention include encouraging comprehensive bans on tobacco advertising, providing pictorial warnings on tobacco products, and providing greater protection from involuntary exposure to tobacco smoke (Collin and Lee 2007). The FCTC is one example of an attempt by WHO to resist unbridled capitalism (McClean 2007).

In sum, we can see the tensions here between public health, trade, the state and globalization. Public health advocates have also attempted to confront health-hostile commercial enterprises by using those enterprises' own marketing strategies.

Fighting Marketing with Marketing

Public health advocates oppose the marketing of certain products but have incorporated commercial marketing techniques to change attitudes and behaviours – known as social marketing. These marketing campaigns are theorized in terms of their mechanisms for changing behaviour – for example, theories of planned behaviour, social cognitive theory and health belief models. Social marketing can include such things as developing a branding strategy for physical activity campaigns – based on the notion that brand affinity creates loyalty. For the VERB™ brand, aimed at encouraging physical activity in 9–13 year olds, advertising agencies like Saatchi and Saatchi were involved (Asbury et al. 2008). The campaigning involved popular athletes, celebrities and cartoon characters in order to build brand equity – the value of the brand (ibid.).

In relation to tobacco control we have a sustained confrontation between multinational companies and public health. Public health has developed campaigns that have the activities of the companies as the focus. In some states in the U.S., media campaigns have highlighted tobacco industry denials about the addictive and harmful nature of its product (Hersey et al. 2005). The names of some anti-tobacco organizations capture this opposition well, such as REBEL – Reaching Everyone By Exposing Lies – in New Jersey (ibid.).

The aim of negative advertising campaigns against corporate tobacco is to reduce trust in the companies (Apollonio and Malone 2009). Public health advocates, in confronting multinational companies, position them as 'disease vectors' and 'disease-promoting industries' (ibid.). Negative advertising campaigns, where messages attack, criticize and discredit corporations, have been shown to be effective in reducing tobacco consumption in teenagers (ibid.). The 'truth' campaign, originally part of a Florida state tobacco-control programme and later taken up by the American Legacy Foundation, was first launched in 1998. It is an example of the use of a social marketing technique, where the brand 'truth®' was developed to compete against tobacco brands and oppose addiction to independence from the tobacco industry (Asbury et al. 2008). 'Truth' was the product in the campaign, as such being opposed to the 'lies' of the tobacco industry. There were a number of negative advertisements created during this campaign, such as the body bags advertisement. In this advertisement teenagers stacked twelve hundred body bags outside the corporate headquarters of Philip Morris, the bags representing the number killed each day by smoking (Apollonio and Malone 2009). Other advertisements attacked corporate irresponsibility, and others highlighted the toxic nature of tobacco.

A number of organizations, such as Adbusters, have been established that promote campaigns of non-cooperation such as 'buy nothing day' (Porter 2008). Adbusters describes itself as 'a global network of culture jammers and creatives working to change the way information flows, the way corporations wield power and the way meaning is produced in our society' (Adbusters, n.d.). Their spoof advertisements parody major food, alcohol and tobacco advertisements.

Sustainability

In the twenty-first century a strong connection has been made in public health between sustainable development and health (Orme et al. 2007b). Public health critiques of trade and commerce go beyond worries about the impact of health-deleterious products to target environment-deleterious activities. Risks to health are articulated in relation to ozone depletion, loss of biodiversity and other forms of environmental degradation that may promote newly emerging diseases, such as SARS (Grey et al. 2007). The concept of sustainability links individual well-being to that of the state of the planet – totalizing the scale of public health. Public health's reach becomes very long indeed when public health and issues of sustainability come into contact. Concepts like sustainable cities and sustainable agriculture can bring together environmental concerns and public health interventions. These concepts are captured in the broader concept of sustainable development where the developments we consider today are undertaken so that they do not damage the health or the environment of future generations (Fudge 2007).

Concerns over sustainability in relation to the forces of production are not new. Marx developed the theoretical concept of metabolic rift that drew attention to concerns about soil fertility in capitalist agricultural production, the pollution of cities, overpopulation and deforestation (Foster 1999). Marx highlighted, for example, the tight association between soil fertility and social relations. Under capitalism, the exploitation of the earth could undermine the conditions of its reproduction (ibid.). The concept of the metabolic rift was a way for Marx to describe the conditions under which the soil would lose its vitality. Under capitalism the industrial population spirals whilst the agricultural population diminishes. The large-scale agricultural production required to feed the industrial populations ruins the soil. The metabolic interaction between people and earth is disrupted. As the worker is alienated the soil is vitiated. Capitalist agriculture disrupts the organic relationship between nature and society. Landowners rob the soil of its nutrients.

The concept of sustainable development, however, gained a particular focus from the 1980 World Conservation Strategy in which sustainable development was viewed as a means of integrating economic development with the maintenance of the environment (Fudge 2007). This view countered alternative views with more radical implications for social organization – that economic growth and the maintenance of the environment were incompatible goals. The context of sustainability is a rapidly growing world population, from an estimated 791 million people in 1750 to 6,055 million in 2000, and an estimated 8,909 million by 2050 (ibid.). Development is also seen as posing a threat to the environment – for example, the number of cars in China grew from 1 million in 1994 to 16 million in 2004 (Scally 2007). Attention to sustainability can invite critiques of trade and commerce. In addition to the 5 million deaths a year caused by tobacco usage, tobacco cultivation has been the cause of the loss of hundreds of thousands of acres of forest annually (ibid.), so tobacco can be criticized for its unsustainability.

The European Commission's understanding of sustainable cities is that developments should not only avoid environmental degradation, but facilitate social equality. Economic prosperity would accompany social inclusion, global sustainability and local empowerment (Fudge 2007). Links between environmental sustainability and individual lifestyle can be made. Contemporary society has been conceptualized as having two plagues of consumption (Scally 2007) – a plague related to overindulgence and a plague related to the unsustainable consumption of the earth's resources. Such concerns clearly link representations of a healthy planet, the health of the population and lifestyles.

The issue of climate change is a unifying concept in relation to sustainability. In 2007, the International Intergovernmental Panel on Climate Change, which was originally set up in 1988 to advise on the risk of climate change, presented the view that changes in the world's climate are without doubt and that human practices have brought these about. In February 2005 the Kyoto Protocol was put in place in an effort to control greenhouse gas emissions. The protocol was negotiated under the auspices of the United Nations Framework Convention on Climate Change.

Public health practitioners have played a role in the development of responses to climate change. One focus has been to identify the possible health impacts of climate change as a way of justifying attempts to respond to the situation. Identified negative health impacts have included those resulting from the spread of vector-borne diseases such as malaria, those resulting from heat waves and other extreme weather events causing a greater death toll, especially amongst the elderly, and those resulting from the follow-on effects of climate change on water and food security (Costello et al. 2009). It would also have indirect impacts through changes to social organization and the economy (Haines et al. 2009). Tools have been developed to assess within-country health impacts of climate change. The tools include the identification of 'climate-sensitive health determinants' (Ebi et al. 2005). The role of public health in responding to climate change is clearly an important and ongoing one.

Like other public health concerns, sustainability can have unusual consequences. For example, it has led to calls to end migration from underdeveloped countries to countries like the U.S., as the migrants' consumption patterns increase to those of the adopted developed country (Labonté 2008).

Discussion

Representations of health inequalities provide a potential rallying point for action and lobbying to bring about policy changes of a radical nature. Radical democracy, redistribution of resources, and a greater focus on equality of outcomes can all be pursued as public health interventions.

Public health draws on many strategies to influence population health that go beyond attempts to influence state and local government. Public health advocacy can directly target particular commercial enterprises whose products can be lethal and whose actions can increase health inequalities. In setting their sights on big corporations, public health advocates may draw on the very same advertising tactics as those corporations use – such as emphasizing brand loyalty and using advertising campaigns.

Public health can also target commerce through international conventions. It can be argued that trade concerns can undermine public health in terms of international agreements with multinational companies using trade agreements against public health efforts. But increasingly public health has taken on an international character, with tobacco covenants being followed by those on climate change, and no doubt public health advocates will pursue a range of other covenants as opportunities arise.

This incredibly wide range of public health activities brings public health into conflict with many institutions, organizations and governments. There are tensions within public health itself, with a focus on lifestyle vying for a focus on social justice at various stages in history and in various jurisdictions. It is perhaps better to see this tension as a productive one rather than an all-out conflict. As will be seen in chapter 4, a focus on lifestyle and risk factor epidemiology allows public health to enter the consultation room, where social justice issues would gain little purchase. But at a national and international level social justice concerns have the potential to influence important policies related to the redistribution of resources and the trading environment.

Public health can come into conflict with the nation-state by confronting governments with the negative health outcomes of policies, yet it can also be enrolled by the nation-state to pursue its objectives – whether those objectives are for the public good, or, as in the case of Nazi Germany, for the pursuit of genocide.

WHO's Commission on Social Determinants of Health had, as one of its principles of action, tackling inequitable power, resource and money distributions (Marmot et al. 2008). Actions to address the social determinants of health are extensive, including fair financing of economic development, gender equity and political empowerment. As the opening of this chapter noted, the Commission's report concluded that 'social injustice is killing people on a grand scale' (CSDH 2008). Combining this powerful rhetoric with the equally powerful imagery that is produced through public health research compellingly leads to the conclusion that some fundamental change in social organization is required to address social injustice.

Public health is in a unique position in contemporary society. It has institutional bases within and outside governments that develop and act on these profound representations of social injustice. Social justice is a principal aspect of Durkheim's cult of humanity, and public health provides collective representations of social justice and injustice, and mechanisms to act on these representations. The next chapter explores the wide reach of public health in the community and some of the challenges in implementing the goal of social justice.

Notes

1. It is not my intention to adjudicate on the claims made by Labonté and others in relation to the role of the IMF. This applies to any 'dispute' or 'controversy' noted in this book. The point, in this instance, is to indicate public health's role in resisting particular social institutions, not to determine whether such a resistance is for the greater good or not.
2. The Cochrane Library contains databases that have been developed to provide independent evidence to inform health care decision making.

CHAPTER 3
Health Promotion Settings and Health Hostile Environments

Introduction

Within the purview of public health, the basic human functions such as drinking, eating and moving are integrated into a system of meaning related to the collective good. While old public health tended to focus on disease, public health in contemporary times has tended to concentrate more on the prevention of chronic illness. The focus on prevention has meant health regimes are no longer limited to the bedridden or the infected. Entire populations are now, potentially, under the scope of initiatives to improve health through their everyday activities. This extension of the clinical gaze has been characterized as surveillance medicine (Armstrong 1983). Often, this is undertaken in the name of empowering the individual. But the concept of empowerment turns out to be something of a contradiction in health promotion, and can be construed to mean obliging individuals to make the appropriate choices as determined by health experts.

Even with surveillance medicine, with its extension to entire populations, there are many population groups within contemporary societies for whom such public health measures have failed to reach, or for whom such measures have been adopted ineffectually. Surveillance medicine has negative connotations, but a lack of surveillance can also have negative consequences.

This chapter will outline the extension of the public health gaze but also the current limitations of public health as surveillance medicine. In particular current limitations will be illustrated in relation to the workplace. There are, of course, many other limitations to the public health gaze. What is of interest about this particular one is the way it illustrates a limitation of public health in relation to capital and business in a particular setting, yet a 'settings approach' to public health has been strongly advocated. Although public health is underpinned by concerns for social justice and empowerment, the lack of penetration in particular sites, such as workplaces, suggests the presence of enduring constraints on public health surveillance. In the case of the workplace setting there is a tension between capital and the profit motive, and the health and safety of workers. Consequently, the health of workers suffers and it is argued here that public health advocacy could play a more meaningful role in relation to vulnerable groups in society, such as workers in health-hostile workplaces. If public health is taking on the mantle of the cult of humanity then its objectives to alleviate suffering and resist health-hostile influences need to extend even further than they have to date.

New Public Health and Health Promotion

As was illustrated in chapter 1, 'old' public health was primarily concerned with acute infectious diseases such as smallpox, cholera and typhoid. Sanitation and vaccination were seen as the means of combating such health hazards. In 'new' public health, particularly in developed countries, there has been a shift to focusing more on chronic diseases – cardiovascular disease and diabetes for instance – and a multiplicity of methods are deployed to change the behaviour of individuals. This is health promotion among populations: encouraging individuals to adopt healthy lifestyles and engage in 'healthy' behaviours, while avoiding those that are said to increase the chances of chronic illness.

Health promotion attempts to change attitudes and behaviours by use of legal, political and mass communication strategies. To some, this is better called health education, as it lends itself to the view that people lack knowledge and therefore experts are required to inform them on how to lead a healthier life. In the past, health education was strongly associated with state paternalism. This is nicely expressed in the views of a government department of health in the 1950s, in the statement that 'the promotion of healthy living then, is our first aim. This is done by education, propaganda, and a little bit of force' (cited in Hyde 1999: 256).

By contrast, others argue that health promotion needs to be underpinned by the goal of empowerment so that people can make their own choices and decisions, and not have to defer to experts (MacDonald 1998). This approach has been strongly linked with the more contemporary 'new public health' (Hyde 1999). In a highly influential statement, the notion and importance of empowerment was forcefully emphasized in the Ottawa Charter 1986. The Ottawa Charter was the outcome of the first international conference on health promotion, and it defines health promotion as a process which enables people to increase control over their own health (Beaglehole 1992). The WHO reiterated this approach with its definition of health promotion as 'the process of enabling people to increase control over, and to improve, their health' (cited in Kendall 1998: 2).

The origins of this notion of empowerment in health promotion discourse can be traced back to feminism and the self-help movements of the 1970s (Kendall 1998). Since the early 1990s, however, the notion has been reframed within a more conservative discourse, so that it is no longer associated with radical collective action but instead is used to assert the importance of individual self-responsibility (ibid.). Models of community health promotion consequently can include concepts of self-empowerment that focus on 'informed choice' but these are seldom able to take account of the external social constraints on those choices. Radical community empowerment models of health promotion can conflict with public health agendas, where, for example, the agenda might be to improve people's healthy choices but inherent in this is a notion of 'wrong' choices (Scambler and Scambler 1998). That is, people may choose practices that are regarded as unhealthy from a public health perspective – and so are making 'bad' decisions.

The larrikin subculture in Australia's Hunter Valley is illustrative of this tension. Health promotion campaigns were implemented in the 1990s to address the higher rates of coronary heart disease in the Coalfields area of the Hunter Valley (Higginbotham et al. 2001). These campaigns, that targeted residents in the area to encourage exercise and low-fat diets, came to nothing. The researchers set out to explore why this was the case, concluding that a complex set of historical and social circumstances fostered a rejection of health messages from experts. A larrikin subculture meant that health promotion messages often failed to penetrate. This culture was one of male solidarity as a way of bolstering working-class masculinity and of retaining dignity while under threat from social discrimination by outsiders. The larrikin response involved a celebration of gambling, drinking and fighting, and meat eating was strongly favoured over low-fat diets as meat was seen as providing strength to those doing hard manual work.

Empowerment is, therefore, a problematic term. Empowerment rhetoric is often deployed in order to achieve compliance with a public health agenda. Information might be provided to individuals but this is in order to ensure that the right choice, the rational choice, the choice that public health experts think is best, is made, and not some other goal such as the pursuit of pleasure or the maintenance of male solidarity. Health promotion therefore faces a paradox in an age where autonomy of the health consumer is given emphasis (MacDonald 1998). How can health promotion both promote individual choice and at the same time convince individuals that the experts know best?

This paradox is illustrated by examples of where efforts to empower people have had the opposite, disempowering effect. In promoting cervical screening programmes certain information about the causes of cervical cancer was disseminated, while other information was not (Hyde 1999). Screening programmes aimed to empower women to take control of their own bodies. But, health promotion campaigns played down the issue of men as transmitters of the virus that can cause cervical cancer. This was done in order to distract from the sexual origins of the disease. Acknowledging the sexual origin of the disease might have dissuaded women from participating in the programme and so this particular piece of information was not given any prominence. The tensions in health promotion between persuasion (or propaganda) and empowerment are clearly revealed.

The work of French theorist Michel Foucault provides a means of making sense of public health and the paradox of empowerment. Foucault argues (Foucault 1978) that over time there have been changes in the way that the individual is produced as a subject that can be understood and managed. As noted in the introduction, from a Foucauldian perspective there has been an increasing emphasis on the biological process of the body. Bodies are understood, and therefore managed, in terms of what is known about their biological composition and physiology. Foucault refers to this as biopower. Foucault argues that we can see this in increasing concerns over birth, mortality, longevity, and all the attention paid by various institutions to the conditions that affect these and other indicators of health amongst individuals and populations. This is the consequence of health regimes that are no longer limited to the bedridden and diseased: with the new public health, entire populations are now potentially under the scope of initiatives to improve health. Foucault argues that biological processes have become regulated through a series of interventions and controls, and thus, so have individuals. The object is to take care of the population and, consequently, as is noted in chapter 1, the state is strengthened (Foucault 1988: 153).

For Foucault, people's lives can be managed and knowledge can be collected via systems of surveillance and the normalization of bodies. Normalization refers to the attempt to make sick or deviant bodies comply with norms of what the body should be and how it should act. It also refers to the process of subjecting the population to standard procedures, such as mass screening and vaccinations (the latter is explored in more detail in chapter 6). Normalization, in other words, can be seen as an attempt to standardize bodies – to make them all the same. By making bodies all the same, and creating a particular self-awareness of the body amongst individuals, people potentially become more compliant and manageable. This allows for greater control or administration of bodies. By subjecting everyone to the same procedures, it becomes easier to identify those who do not conform, and therefore to develop strategies to coerce or force people to comply with the objectives of public health.

David Armstrong (1983) argues that this clinical gaze extended to a much broader population in the interwar years in England. This was brought about by the findings of the 'Peckham Experiment', which began in 1935 and became the rationale for establishing the National Health Service (NHS). The experiment involved the establishment of the Pioneer Health Centre in the London suburb of Peckham. The centre was open to any family living within a mile (or walking distance). Families would pay one shilling a week subscription to become members, and would have access to the club and its equipment, which included a swimming pool, gymnasium and a billiard table. Members would also be subject to periodic health assessments (Pearse and Crocker 1947). During the course of the experiment, it was determined that the 'treatable' population was much larger than expected. Of the first five hundred families subjected to the health overhaul it was found that 31.6 per cent of family members had some disorder that was accompanied by disease, and another 59 per cent appeared to be well but had some underlying problem that should receive some sort of therapeutic intervention. A mere 9 per cent of the population were therefore regarded as healthy. It was concluded that care should also be directed at those not yet born:

> In existing circumstances the consecutive care of the infant only begins after its birth, whereas it has been growing from the moment of conception. Neither is there any provision whereby the advantages of modern medical science can become available to all potential and prospective parents before conception, so ensuring that the child shall inherit its birthright of health. (Pearse and Crocker 1947: 11)

This was, then, a justification for initiating a range of practices which, in effect, brought about the extension of the clinical gaze. Health professions expanded their focus from the treatment of disease to its prevention, a greater proportion of the population became subjected to health care, and medicine further infiltrated the lives of individuals (Armstrong 1983). Almost the entire population, and many areas of an individual's life, could then be drawn into the web of biopower.

The extension of the clinical gaze has become increasingly entwined with technological and managerial systems. Computerized registers and automatic call-ups for patients, for instance, allow for standardized and ordered management of information on the bodies of a population. Power over people, then, is intensified as information about them is incorporated into new technologies that facilitate the control of the population.

Foucault suggests that as we gain more knowledge about bodies and how bodies interact with the social and physical environment, then individuals are increasingly subjected to the effects of power. As knowledge of the body has been produced, and practices have been put in place to eradicate abnormalities, individuals become subject to power. We are, in a sense, produced, moulded and restricted by the technologies and knowledge that we aim to use to improve our health. We come to know ourselves, and our bodies, in a particular way, and we consequently come to engage in certain activities, while refraining from others. In the name of health, means have been developed to increasingly discipline our lives from birth to death. From the needle-prick screening when a baby is born to our hospitalized deaths, we are described, prescribed and regulated. But it is not simply that these regimes of power, as Foucault calls them, are imposed upon us. We impose them upon ourselves, and even demand them. Thus, 'empowerment' can be seen to be constructed out of a desire for regulation and prescription.

However, despite the influence of public health and its various practices and measures aimed at producing good, healthy citizens, we need to avoid considering public health developments as monolithic, uncontainable and all encompassing. Foucault argues that wherever there is power, there is counter-power, struggle and resistance. The larrikin culture is but one illustration of this. New procedures of power over the body lead to new forms and instances of political struggle (Foucault 1978). Power is not something that is held by a particular group of elites, it is, rather, the effect of relations, and since relations are changeable and unstable, perhaps even reversible, so is power. There is, then, the potential to challenge and reconfigure all power relations (McNay 1992).

Setting and Extending Health Promotion

Since the Peckham Experiment, further means to deepen and extend the clinical gaze have been developed through health promotion activities. Mechanisms to enhance public health activities have included developing concepts like the 'obesogenic environment' and mechanisms for enrolling all sectors in public health activities like health impact assessments and healthy public policy. These will be discussed in chapter 7. The concept of settings and community participation, discussed here, also extend the gaze.

In relation to a settings approach in health promotion, Fleming (2007: 167) describes a setting as 'any defined entity, organization or geographical area where a whole system approach can be adopted to the improvement of health at both the individual and population level'. Settings have also been described as 'the domains of the living environment, the working environment and the leisure/cultural environment' (Orme et al. 2007b: 19). According to this view, any city, neighbourhood, workplace, school or space in which people come together can act as a setting that can be a space of health promotion.

A broad-based settings approach could be seen in the Health Action Zone (HAZ) initiatives in England, which lasted from 1998 to 2003 under New Labour. HAZs were multi-agency partnerships that aimed to improve health and reduce inequalities in deprived areas of England. HAZ projects focused on the determinants of health and local health service delivery. There were twenty-six HAZs established, from the relatively small, such as Luton with a population of 200,000, to the large, such as Merseyside with a population of 1.4 million. One-third of the initial programmes were aimed at tackling issues related to the determinants of health such as employment, housing and education (Bauld and Mackenzie 2007). There were seven principles underlying HAZ; achieving equity, engaging communities, working in partnership, engaging front-line staff, taking an evidence-based approach, developing a person-centred approach to service delivery, and taking a whole-systems approach. For example, as it was known that low-income smokers were less likely to use cessation services and that their quit rates were lower, these disadvantaged groups could be targeted through HAZ (Amos 2007). But the outcomes for health inequalities were ambiguous. In relation to smoking, quit rates remained lower for the disadvantaged, however the services met proportionately more of them – so possibly contributing to the lessening of inequalities.

Tobacco reduction strategies are a clear example where the outcomes of public health interventions have the potential to further exacerbate health inequalities. In the U.K. there was an overall reduction in cigarette smoking between 1974 and 1984, but the gap between the smoking rates of the advantaged and the disadvantaged actually increased. This was due to the fact that approaches to reduce smoking were more effective for those who were more affluent than for the more deprived. Inequalities were not reduced between these groups, even though there was a drop in smoking rates for all groups (Amos

2007). Amos points out that the strategy of raising tobacco taxes as a means of reducing smoking rates hits the low socioeconomic groups the hardest – who also may find it the most difficult to quit. Increasing prices can also encourage smuggling, and 'smuggled tobacco products are particularly prevalent in deprived areas' (Amos 2007: 198). The danger with smuggling is that the quality of cigarettes cannot be guaranteed, and so counterfeits can be more damaging to health.

Another example of an expansive settings approach is the Healthy Cities initiative. In 1987 WHO founded the Healthy Cities Programme, which aimed to 'provide an effective means of dealing with health-related aspects of poverty, pollution, lifestyle changes, urban planning, transport and the special needs of marginalized and vulnerable groups in urban areas' (Lawrence and Fudge 2007: 180). Principles underpinning Healthy Cities include 'control by the public over the decisions affecting their lives' and a 'non-exploitive' community (ibid.: 184). The latter is based on equity, implying 'a just distribution of the benefits and services in a society with respect to a universal standard of values such as human rights' (ibid.). A strong underpinning of social justice is evident in these approaches.

Schools are a good example of the extension of health promotion into smaller settings. Schools have been regarded by government agencies as a delivery mechanism for tackling health inequalities (Pike and Colquhoun 2009) as well as a way of attending to the 'obesity epidemic' (Porter 2008). They have been the focus for educating about health, increasing physical activity and improving nutrition. In relation to the latter, attempts have been made to introduce meals to schools, so that children from poor backgrounds can be adequately fed and so potentially take better advantage of school education (Pike and Colquhoun 2009). Nutrition guidelines have also been developed to stipulate what types of food can be served at schools.

Powerful justifications for focusing on the earlier years of life, rather than adult health, come from a variety of sources. Early years of development are thought to play a crucial role in reproducing health inequalities. The early years of life are thought to establish the basis of health behaviours and health outcomes in later life (Li et al. 2009). So not only do schools become a focus, but pre-school is increasingly seen as an important stage for health intervention.

This thinking has led to the development of programmes to intervene early in childhood, such as the Sure Start and Head Start programmes. Sure Start in the U.K., announced in 1997, was directed at pre-school children and their families in disadvantaged areas. This was part of a 'social inclusion' strategy. Projects included home visiting programmes, early child care programmes and health care programmes. The initiative was directed towards the upstream provision of services, which are prevention and early intervention focused, as opposed to downstream provision such as acute and restorative services. In the U.S., their Head Start and High/Scope programmes, based on similar goals, date back to the 1960s.

Sure Start was based around universal access to services within particular 'deprived' geographical areas. Evaluation of Sure Start revealed, however, that those in the community with more resources were the ones accessing the services, and as a consequence those who were more disadvantaged might not be able to access those services, so having a negative impact on the latter (Gidley 2007). This illustrates a particular difficulty in public health and health promotion, which is that vulnerable groups either do not respond to interventions or, as in this case, have a negative outcome as a result of the intervention. Conversely, the already privileged gain further benefits.

Evaluation of health promotion activities in schools suggests they are also variable in what they achieve (Pike and Colquhoun 2009). In contrast to planned health promotion activities, King argues that 'Jamie's School Dinners', a popular U.K. television series screened in 2005 which drew attention to the 'appalling state of school meals in the U.K.', led to a public outcry and government pressure that public health practitioners had not been able to achieve (King 2007). This could be read as demonstrating the weakness of traditional public health advocacy – all it takes to get some action is to get a celebrity doing the job. But it also demonstrates how celebrities and programme producers can take on a public health agenda.

Scriven (2007) suggests that new forms of health activism have developed in relation to celebrity status. Besides Jamie Oliver, Bill Gates and pop musicians have also undertaken activist roles. But this use of celebrities for health promotion has attracted criticism. Examples of popular politics, such as the 'make poverty history' celebrity campaigns, have been condemned by some public health advocates for their shallowness in failing to take into consideration the global dynamics of debt and poverty (Labonté 2008).

Community Participation

Engaging communities has been an important principle of health promotion approaches. Involving communities in health development and social regeneration programmes is now a requirement of many British government strategies to tackle health inequalities. This can be based around the concept of social capital as a buffer to socio-economic disadvantage (Morgan and Popay 2007). Social capital, as a term, was first coined in 1916, and has come to mean, in public health, 'shared understandings, levels of trust, associational memberships and informal networks of human relationships that facilitate social exchange, social order and underpin social institutions' (Richardson and Mumford cited in Gilchrist 2007). Morgan and Popay argue that social capital is seen as a resource for societies, and where social capital is high then so is trust and community life. Programmes in the U.K. have been explicitly based on the idea that increased social interaction would have a positive impact on people's health (Morgan and Popay 2007). So not only do our personal daily activities of breathing, eating and moving come into the public health orbit, but also the relationships we have with those around us, near and far.

Responses to the findings of the Peckham Experiment also brought about a focus on social capital and related concepts. In the U.K., the development of

Healthy Living Centres, which facilitate activities for patients and community participation as a preventive function of public health, is regarded as having its roots in the Peckham Experiment (Gilchrist 2007). Community participation, in and of itself, is seen as beneficial for public health. This notion is central to Durkheim's concerns in relation to social solidarity and connectedness in modern society.

The concept of social capital became prominent in public health discourse in the 1990s. However, it has been argued that, far from being a means of tackling inequalities, the focus on the role of civic organizations and community action provided by the concept of social capital fits with political ideologies linked to minimizing the role of the state in addressing health inequalities (Green and Labonté 2008a). Following this view, a focus on participation and engagement could distract from structural issues like a lack of material resources or the need for greater redistribution of resources.

Additionally, public health interventions to enhance communities that are 'hard to reach' can have ambiguous outcomes in relation to community participation and social capital. This is nicely illustrated in Singleton's analysis of the Community Heart Care Initiative in north-west England (Singleton 2005). This initiative was an outcome of what has been termed the 'new public health' which positions healthy citizens as active, competent and skilled members of their own community (ibid.). The aim of the initiative was to train all members of the community in cardio-pulmonary resuscitation (CPR), train members of the public in the use of defibrillators which were placed in public spaces such as railway stations, and develop a 'first responder' scheme where members of the community would carry defibrillators in case of an emergency. The latter aimed to address the problem of the time it can take for a paramedic to arrive in the case of a member of the public suffering a heart attack. This initiative relates to the health promotion concepts of empowerment and the goal of fostering social capital.

Singleton's research reveals the moral categories that permeate interventions such as these, which attempt to foster good citizenship. Non-participants were characterized as 'couch potatoes' and 'ignorant', whereas participants were constructed as caring and good. Non-participants were regarded as lacking in humanity and neighbourliness. But not everyone could claim the moral high ground. To be a first responder one needed a car. And for some the lack of training could lead to guilt if they were not able to intervene successfully in the case of a heart attack. Singleton cites a case of the guilt over not undertaking CPR training from the wife of an 80-year-old who died from a heart attack (Singleton 2005). This guilt is 'promoted' in such interventions, perhaps unwittingly, even though it is known that CPR saves few lives.

The goals of empowerment through health promotion may be elusive. Public health interventions may be implemented, but with little effect or with unforeseen outcomes. The clinical gaze and the web of biopower may have spread to many areas of life, and much of the population, but there are nevertheless numerous instances, even within the developed world, where public health has failed to infiltrate.

Hard-to-Reach Groups

Settings approaches extend health promotion in many different directions with some anticipated and some unanticipated consequences. However, even with this extension, there are still many groups that remain outside the purview of public health and health promotion. For example, it has been argued that disabled people are currently excluded from public health practice (Watson 2007). At the clinical level this includes GPs providing less health promotion advice to patients with mental health problems, and people with learning difficulties being less likely to receive health checks. Public health tends to prioritize conditions which have an impact on large numbers in the population, such as diabetes, heart disease and cancers. This is in line with the health economics principle of efficiency, as it is these conditions that cost the most money and, by implication, provide the possibility of making the most savings if the burden of disease can be reduced (Forman 2008). Conversely, rare diseases, including neurological conditions and metabolic disorders, get little attention in relation to public health priorities and action. The calls from the WHO and other agencies to orient services away from clinical and curative services to health promotion and preventative services, exacerbates this issue. Unless they happen to be the focus of genetic screening (such as those aimed at identifying cystic fibrosis or phenylketonuria), rare diseases are usually dealt with at the clinical level, not the preventative level (ibid.).

This lack of prioritization for rare conditions also affects research. Public health research has a greater chance of securing funding if it focuses on major diseases. The messages are often contradictory in relation to research, revealing a tension between economic efficiency and social justice: on the one hand a utilitarian argument appears to be made, and on the other, a social justice concern to reach marginalized and vulnerable groups. Funding applications for health research clearly reveal this contradiction. For the New Zealand Health Research Council applications, one-quarter of the assessment score in the scientific committees is determined by health significance, that is, the impact that the research is likely to have on health outcomes. The Australian National Health and Medical Research Council claims commitment to advancing Aboriginal and Torres Strait Islander health research. But again, research is to have significant outcomes. The construct of 'significance' is suggestive of outcomes that will have a big impact – which is much harder to achieve if the focus is on a numerically minor group. On this basis, conditions that impact upon the majority of the population, such as diabetes and cardiovascular disease, will score higher. Rare diseases, however debilitating, will score lower, as will research that does not include the majority of the population.

An illustration of this tension is revealed in a 'Request for Proposals' on interventions in primary care and public health settings, which states that 'The workplace setting is advantageous to health promotion, due to but not limited to ease of access to a large number of people'. This is, in essence, a utilitarian argument supporting the most efficient use of available resources. Later in the form it states that 'research should look at the application of primary care in workplace settings, with a particular focus on "hard to engage" populations'. This is a social justice argument – however, such hard to engage or marginalized groups are likely to be overrepresented in small factories and workplaces where there is very little union representation or public health reach, rather than bigger workplace settings. The utilitarian and social justice arguments are clearly in opposition.

Hard-to-Reach Workplaces

It is notable that the language of empowerment used in public health initiatives at the community or neighbourhood level – getting communities to make decisions about their own environment and so on – is absent in public health initiatives related to the workplace. Fleming points out that a challenge within workplace settings is the health promotion concept of empowerment in a situation where there are structural power imbalances (Fleming 2007). Public health and health promotion would confront strong ideological positions if attempts were made to introduce worker empowerment as a public health measure. Worker empowerment has the flavour of socialism and a radical reorganization of the workplace.

Currently there are initiatives to promote healthier eating and more active lifestyles in the workplace (Allender et al. 2006), but these are directed at influencing individual behaviours. Health promotion workplace initiatives tend to take a different focus from empowerment. In the U.K., the Healthy Workplace Initiative was designed to improve health and reduce inequalities in health. Initiatives included assisting workers who fall ill 'to re-enter the workplace as quick [*sic*] as possible' (Fleming 2007: 174) and work-life balance campaigns. Neither of these provides any fundamental challenge to social organization.

Public health researchers with a focus on the workplace have been criticized for focusing on workers who are accessible rather than on those most in need (Polanyi et al. 2008). The focus of research is influenced by research funders and compensation schemes; so, for example, those who are not covered by compensation schemes, such as illegal workers, are not prioritized in health research (ibid.). The area of occupational health research has been accused, as Daykin suggests, of serving 'the interests of employers at the expense of workers: by minimizing the scale of work-related illness; limiting the protection of health; ignoring and devaluing workers' experience of occupational ill health and focusing on individual behavior in explaining work-related illness' (1999: 7).

Health promotion in the workplace is based on the notion that benefits will accrue to workers as a result of improved health and safety, increased job satisfaction and other factors (Fleming 2007). Benefits for employers include reduced turnover and absenteeism (ibid.). Institutional centres for this approach include the European Network of Health Promoting Workplaces (ENHPW). The ENHPW subordinates its goals to 'social and economic success in Europe' through the implementation of workplace health promotion (ibid.: 167).

Adkins suggests that health promotion activities in the workplace, which focus on the lifestyle of the worker, are an extension of surveillance medicine (Adkins 2002: 29). Although not denying this, there is in fact a lack of surveillance in many workplaces that makes invisible a range of practices that are detrimental to health. In chapter 5, the impact of surveillance medicine in further disempowering vulnerable workers will be addressed; however, the argument presented here focuses on the opposite issue. That is, where a lack of surveillance by public health in the workplace can make workers vulnerable to hazards and prone to health problems. This sounds like a contradiction – but it simply reflects the diverse roles and impacts that public health has in complex environments.

The Anomic Workplace Environment

This section draws on research of worker health and well-being (Dew et al. 2005b; Dew and Taupo 2009). Not all workplaces are hostile to health and there are obvious health-enhancing features of work. But work environments that are 'health hostile' are not difficult to find. These problematic workplaces that elude the reach of public health can be made sense of with Durkheim's two types of pathological forms of the division of labour (ibid.). For Durkheim, problems arise from either an absence of regulation (anomie) on one level, or coercive regulation (forced division of labour) on another. In the anomic division of labour a lack of regulation results in an increase in competition and class conflict. A lack of regulation may involve unrestricted competition or an absence of agreement over the regulation of prices and incomes. In the second form, a forced or coercive division of labour, the rules of the division of labour are inherently unjust and so solidarity between individuals will not materialize. An example would be an irregularity of opportunities for particular social groups (Thompson 1982). This situation could be changed if the state took a more decisive role in securing the conditions under which individuals could develop their potential.

Such problematic workplaces will be shown in the following illustrations; there is an absence of regulation regarding health, or if there are regulations, they are either inadequate or not adhered to; health and well-being are also compromised by enforced divisions of labour, disempowering workers; and there is a clear tension between capitalism, or the profit imperative, and the health and well-being of workers.

Both large and small workplaces can be hostile environments, lacking the emphasis on health and well-being that underlies public health. Workers can face extremely hostile health environments, even in developed countries, and workers can have very little choice in relation to the working conditions they have to deal with (Dew et al. 2005b).

The distance between the ideals of health promotion and the lived experience of workplace settings is evident in the conditions of a small factory. The health of workers may be overridden in order to ensure the manufactured product is maintained at the correct temperature. In certain parts of the factory heaters are supplied 'because they need them in there for the [product], and the rest of the place is freezing cold ... their policy is you don't worry about the workers ... the [product] is their most important thing' (ibid.). This particular factory is always noisy and dangerous, with accounts of workers getting limbs caught in the machinery and of spindles flying from some machines.

For workers in this environment there is very little sense of choice or empowerment. They are isolated from other work sites, and at a time when unions have been fighting for survival, workers at small sites have had little representation. In such 'settings', health promotion activities are absent, and public health measures of a traditional type would seem to have little impact on the health of workers. The hazardous working conditions are more important to the immediate health of workers than exercise and dieting programmes that might be promoted. Such examples suggest that productivity and efficiency take precedence over the health and welfare of workers. In such circumstances workers are not so much rendered as biological and physiological entities, who are thus encouraged to engage in certain healthy living activities; rather, they are configured as and reduced to instrumental components in a larger set of operations, driven by a profit-imperative.

Research conducted in a meat-processing plant illustrates the anomic workplace, highlighting the negative health impact of external market influences on the workplace, the hazardous environment of the workplace, problems with enforcing safety measures, and the role played by company doctors (see Dew and Taupo 2009, for an extended discussion of this example). When workers were asked to describe their working conditions they generally tended to outline concerns that ranged from the big heavy-duty machinery they negotiated and slippery floors, to the dramatic increase in the speed at which meat was required to be cut to meet market demand.

Workers often expressed their frustration about market demand being the driving force and influence on the speed of the cuts and the density of the work. As a result, many workers felt they were treated like machines rather than people: 'Yeah, they've just got to forget about the company sometimes and think about us as individual people not just whatever machines, 'cause we're not machines'.

From the workers' perspective, external market forces are a context for both the pace of work and the way in which workers feel they are treated. Workers talked of being locked in behind machines, making it difficult to exit if there were to be an emergency. One worker provided an account of injuring her back whilst blocked in between a wall and the machine. The company doctor was alerted but did not attend. Workers tried to manoeuvre the worker out of the confined space. As she recounted the experience: '[the] workers ... were really good when I got injured. [They] were the ones who actually got me out of that area, the supervisor didn't even bother. All he wanted to do was keep the production [going] on.'

Risks from knives and equipment were described: 'the belt, you go and duck under, you can get a crack on the head'. Workers raised many other concerns about the conditions of work, including exposure to meal and coal dust, floors made slippery with congealed blood, uncontrolled stock, the dangers of contracting diseases from stock such as leptospirosis, and long working hours during busy times in the season.

Long hours could result from loyalty to colleagues and the workplace, with some workers claiming 'it's nothing for us to do 24 hours'. Workers accrued a variety of work injuries such as cuts, burns, swollen arms and legs due to performing repetitive tasks, and back injuries caused by standing for long periods or from falls. Sometimes, workers were injured due to their efforts when trying to contain animals:

> Well, the goats go through the gates … I went to catch his head and grab him, and he spun around and opened my hand up.

Processing the animals could also be hazardous:

> Yeah, I had this done, a few vertebras out in my neck up there on the chain, the head cutters, where they get heads cut off, when the head gets cut off you can usually push them down with your hand. One of those days it was blunt and I gave it a huge push down, you know what it's like when you kick something that isn't there, your leg goes beyond its reach or whatever … My spine just went crack, crack, crack … and I slipped a disc on it and it pressed the nerves.

Tombs and Whyte argue that pursuing safety in the workplace can place firms at a competitive disadvantage (Tombs and Whyte 2007). As has been well documented elsewhere (Dew 1999b; Wynne 1987), and discussed further in chapter 5, when safety measures are introduced in workplaces, as laid down by experts, they are not always met. The reality of the work situation means that many of the safety measures can be unfeasible, and can cause additional difficulties for workers. Workers may avoid wearing hats because they are too heavy and cause headaches. When asked if she wore her protective gear one worker responded:

> When I want to. Like I can go and bone out a carcass or something [and] the supervisor can walk past and I've got no mesh apron on. There [is] no enforcement. [For instance] someone got cut really bad, on their stomach a woman in our boning room got cut on her stomach, she wasn't wearing a mesh apron either, she was only trimming, and I think they sort of made people wear their mesh aprons after that but it faded away. People stopped wearing them; go in there now and hardly anyone wears them.

Government health and safety representative visits were generally reactive in terms of health and safety policy. Workers stated that when health and safety inspectors carried out their general inspections the workers were not questioned about any health and safety concerns.

For many of the workers the company doctor regularly presented himself as the gatekeeper to wellness. Access to compensation and support by management seemed to be determined by the response of the company doctor. Worker engagement with the company doctor was often challenging and difficult. This is illustrated in the following extensive quote about an incident following the severance of a finger. The quote also exemplifies the extreme, hazardous situations faced by some workers:

> I went in to do the cut and my hand went with the carcass and yeah, went off ... I just got someone to cover me and I went to the office, told the boss and he flipped out, and then we went over, come over to first aid, and [the doctor] looked at it and then sat in the office and talked to my foreman ... and left me sitting out there, he didn't even put my finger on ice. He did nothing. And I was just left there to wait for the ambulance. I had to hold it up and apply pressure to it with a towel, but to me that wasn't the problem ... even the ambulance women and the doctors at the hospital said that finger could have been saved, could have had it back if he had done what he had suppose to do, but it just, I use to think the world of working for this company, but I don't cause it treated me like a carcass ... This one has to come off cause it can't bend, and ... any little bang it hurts, if this gets whacked the whole hand hurts. I still have trouble with it, if it's too cold it's just pain that shoots up my arm, but you get over it, you get used to it. I lost the small finger and this one had to be reconstructed because I nearly just about cut this one off and this one here they sewed that one up, sew the tendons.

The company doctor also administered cortisone on a regular basis to workers who complained of arm, shoulder, wrist, back or leg pain. Some workers did not want to seek medical advice from the company doctor as this often presented more problems for the workers. Following an injury, workers reported being pressured by the company doctor to return to work prematurely:

> It was only with [the company doctor]. I came in to see him because I had a wire that was sticking out of my finger here ... I came to see [the company doctor] for a check up and he wanted me to start back at work with the wire still in it. I just went off my nut ... And I went to see my surgeon ... and told him and he said that I had to ignore [the company doctor].

Failure to return to work could result in wage loss or job loss. In many instances workers would return to their old working area and perform another job. This was referred to as light duties. However, for some workers light duties amounted to intense work similar to their regular work.

One employee complained of suffering severe soreness and pain, but this was dismissed by the company doctor. As a result the employee sought advice from his own doctor who confirmed he had the serious disease leptospirosis. Leptospirosis is a particular workplace risk for meatworkers, who make up nearly 50 per cent of all recorded cases of the disease in New Zealand (Keenan 2007). The company doctor still ignored recommendations made by other experts. This left the employee frustrated and angry after working twelve years for the company and never having been on compensation:

> The company doctor didn't want to know about my illness so he just sent me back to work and everything. So I went to my own doctor and he goes that's a serious thing that's wrong with you … I went into hospital for over a week 'cause both my kidneys shut down and I was spewing up dried blood, it took the specialist over there to do all the tests. And I had lepto, they confirmed it was lepto and I brought all the papers back to the company doctor and the doctor still didn't want to have anything to do with the specialist paper, nothing. And still he tried to blame something else. He won't recognize it as being lepto from the freezing works, but it is.
>
> Interviewer: *What's he saying it's from?*
>
> He's saying stupid things like, he'll say 'for all we know you could have caught lepto from when a rat bit you' and how stupid it that, that's how he talks to you … yeah, he's trying to make it a non-work thing, that's his job I suppose, I've had hell, they didn't want to pay me for eight weeks, I had no money for eight weeks and I was going mad. I had a hell of a time with them. Still do now.

These examples so far are illustrations of what could be conceived of as a lack of regulation and adequate safety measures in the work place. There are also numerous instances where health and well-being are under threat from the enforced division of labour. Such forms of coercion are obstacles to solidarity and empowerment. Workers, for instance, have had to cope with managers who verbally abuse them as they set about their tasks. When asked if they could identify any issues that impacted on their mental health or well-being, one worker relayed the following incident: 'The supervisor stresses us out. He calls us can I swear? black bitches, Abbo's … because I've told him if he calls me a black bitch or Abbo I'll hit him. And I've told the union and the union delegate I will hit him, I don't care if I lose my job.'

Another manifestation of the forced division of labour creating divisions between groups was an ethnic division of labour where indigenous Mäori workers were mainly in manual labour roles whilst workers of European descent were in management roles.

Many of these issues were exacerbated by the pressure to stay at work, despite sickness or exhaustion. Sometimes the pressure stemmed from anxiety passed on by fellow colleagues who would have to pick up the slack for their absent workmate. Participants were also concerned about the impact of not having income to support families whilst ill or injured. Peer pressure from colleagues was also an issue. A worker who contracted leptospirosis said colleagues looked at him 'sideways'. Another worker claimed that the works was not a healthy environment and that some workers wanted to leave 'because people [they] started with 18 years ago are [now] unhealthy or dead'. However, due to economic dependency regarding mortgages and children, they are forced to stay in the job. For many workers interviewed, then, the preferred choice was to work while sick or injured due to economic and social constraints, especially where young children were concerned. After severing a finger and damaging another, one worker stated that she really needed to be at work as the financial burden was too much: 'I come to work because I've got kids to feed. I do it for my kids to give them an education. But if I had a choice, I wouldn't be here.'

These examples illustrate just how fraught the workplace can be. Access to compensation is not necessarily straightforward, and requires the mandate of a company doctor who, as these examples suggest, does not always prioritize the health and well-being of workers. Dwyer (1991) notes that medical doctors in industrial plants commonly submit to the demands of employers or ensure they practice in ways that are compatible with employer interests.

Such workplaces, then, represent settings where public health measures have failed to infiltrate with much success. When safety measures have been adopted, they can be cumbersome, interfering with the comfort and the efficiency of workers, and are therefore often ignored. In these work environments, the imperative to be efficient and productive hinders efforts to encourage healthy living.

One way of articulating the disturbing lack of attention to the health and safety of workers is through the concept of safety crimes. Tombs and Whyte argue that new trends in the workplace are placing workers in more hazardous situations. These trends include the increase in the number of workers in temporary or insecure jobs, 'meaner' welfare systems, and the requirement to work longer, harder and faster (Tombs and Whyte 2007). Combined, these put pressure on workers to stay in jobs that might be hazardous and diminish the scope for resistance to unsafe work practices. Despite these pressures, 'safety crimes' are relatively invisible at the popular and political level. What Tombs and Whyte call safety crimes are often viewed as accidents, disasters and tragedies – and not crimes for which any person or organization is accountable.

Tombs and Whyte provide a number of examples of safety crimes that led to death and injury to workers. An astounding example of a safety crime is the Bhopal disaster of 1984, when an industrial accident at a Union Carbide pesticide manufacturing plant sent poisonous gases into the air. It has been estimated that there were over seven thousand deaths as a direct consequences of this, and around one hundred thousand survivors were not able to work again (Tombs and Whyte 2007). The impact of this particular safety crime went way beyond the factory workforce. The International Labour Organization estimates that there are at least 2.2 million deaths per year as a result of workplace accidents or disease (ibid.). Within the U.K. it has been estimated that there are over ten thousand deaths every year as a result of work-related medical conditions (Slapper and Tombs 1999). This suggests that there is some institutional problem here – some lack of a mediating agency between workers, employers and the state to respond adequately to the health and safety of workers.

One important mediating agency in the workplace is the workers' union. Unions have been accused of having more of a focus on wage negotiations than on workplace safety, although at times unions have been major players in introducing health and safety regulations, such as within the mining and textile industries. Tombs and Whyte suggest that different attitudes to unions can have different outcomes in terms of worker safety, contrasting anti-trade unionism in the U.K. with rights for unions in Norway in terms of the safety records of their respective offshore oil industries. Tombs and Whyte suggest that we need to think beyond simple deterrence to provide better incentives to protect workers. We need to look at the conditions that give rise to the crime rather than simply focusing on the punishment of the criminal – that is, to develop a political economy approach to safety crimes. As they suggest, this includes the research-based view that strong trade union representation provides for safer workplaces. But also that there need to be ways of making management more accountable for decisions. In addition, workers and the public can provide collective opposition to safety crimes, and alternative means of avoiding worker deaths need to be sought.

Dwyer argues that historically the union movement has not concentrated on accidents, leaving this responsibility to site-based safety committees, focusing instead on compensation issues. But a weak union movement does not facilitate worker protection. For example, he points out that in the U.S. sixty thousand lives were lost in the coal-mining sector between 1910 and 1940 but no federal laws were passed in relation to this issue in this period, a time of a weakened union movement. The mere presence of unions does not reduce accidents. In order to achieve this, unions need to increase the workers' collective strength and voice in relation to safety issues. But Dwyer also notes that workers themselves may not always be best placed to reduce accidents – workers may take little interest in accident reduction if the reward structure at work promotes a faster pace of work and so on.

Any particular worksite is situated within global networks that impact upon the role of unions. Bauman argues that liquid modernity has replaced a Fordist heavy or solid modernity – with a new emphasis on flexibility, individuality and choice (Bauman 2000). For Bauman, capital can travel fast and light in liquid or fluid modernity, but labour cannot. As such labour is deprived of its bargaining power and immobilized (ibid.).

Bauman notes that present day uncertainty in work is a powerful individualizing force leading to an incapacity for workers to find common cause. Therefore union action becomes inadequate. If Bauman's reading is right then unions are not well placed to alleviate the misery of the workers. Wills and Hales note that in an environment of networked capitalism where multinational companies subcontract production and can reconfigure supply chains in situations where unions organize for better pay and working conditions, then 'organizing at the workplace is no longer enough' (Wills and Hales 2005: 7). According to Wills and Hales, this new configuration requires transnational solidarity between workers and consumers – and they point to examples like Women Working Worldwide and anti-sweat shop activists in North America. Tombs and Whyte, who take a Gramscian approach to corporate crime, argue that the state and corporations often have a symbiotic relationship, and that it is in the interests of the powerful that certain activities 'be as invisible and remain as absent from the public gaze and scrutiny as possible' (Tombs and Whyte 2003: 4).

Given all these structural factors that inhibit the activities of unions, it is argued here that public health can act as a health promoting force that is external to the workplace, to temper the health-threatening nature of other external forces that currently predominate. Public health can act on the world stage to promote worker health, and thus an international public health approach would not be immobilized in the way that labour is. Dwyer argues that there is a need for a sociologically informed school of accident prevention but he is not clear on who could act in this capacity – and the analysis I am suggesting proffers a sociologically informed public health as a candidate.

Discussion

Public health in the workplace has tended to focus on individual behaviours rather than directing attention to the potential negative impacts of unregulated capitalism on the safety of workers. However, health promotion at the workplace could emphasize such issues as the control that workers have over their work processes, and the capacity of workers to resist hazardous demands from management. The linking of industrial and public health concerns can play an important role in bringing about legislative reform of workplaces. For example, linking particular workplace practices in the cotton industry to concerns about tuberculosis played a vital part in reforming hazardous workplace practices in the cotton industry in the twentieth century (Dale et al. 2007). As such, public health has a rich legacy to call upon, but in developed countries it has resiled from a social justice approach in workplaces.

An obligation under the United Nations 1966 International Covenant on Economic, Social and Cultural Rights is to improve all aspects of industrial hygiene and prevent occupational diseases (Beaglehole and Bonita 1997). Beaglehole and Bonita argue that such statements have important symbolic value for public health professionals in pointing out equity as a goal for public health. They note that occupational hazards are more likely to be faced by workers in poor countries. Public health needs to strive to develop a broad perspective with a focus on socio-structural inequalities in health and not a narrow focus on individual risks of disease. The argument being made in relation to the material presented in this chapter is that public health should also focus on an intermediate 'institutional' level. This is not to lessen the need for public health to contribute to broader policy level discussions on social inequality – but to consider practical tools of intervention at the level of the workplace.

The workplace is not the only setting where health promotion activities are constrained and limited. Public health in prisons would be another settings approach reaching vulnerable groups – but there is very little evidence of prisons being a public health focus.

An important caveat on any call to enhance health promotion activities is the need to be alert to potential unintended outcomes of such activities. Singleton's analysis signals ways in which new identities and moralities can be constructed as an outcome of health promotion programmes aimed at 'empowering' people.

Public health is paradoxical. It is a form of disciplinary power, but if expanded to certain settings it has the potential to play an important role in protecting the vulnerable. A critical task of public health is to identify and attend to the marginal, hard to reach and vulnerable in the knowledge that this further extends surveillance medicine.

We must be alert to the ways in which knowledge is produced, conveyed and suppressed and what impact this exerts on our lives. This analysis, drawing on both Foucault and Durkheim, attends to both the positive and negative aspects of public health and health promotion, but also highlights the importance of a critical analysis of health initiatives, where we look for the effects of power. To link the work of Foucault to Durkheim, we can argue here that Foucault orients us to the construction and effects of power, and Durkheim to the institutional requirements to temper those effects.

CHAPTER 4
Public Health and Health Professionals

Introduction

In schools of public health you will find, perhaps lurking at the end of the corridor or placed on a different floor from her epidemiological colleagues, a health economist. Health economics has become an integral part of public health, and when the procedures of economic calculation are married to epidemiological descriptions, something quite potent is produced. With their utilitarian underpinnings, these two forms of quantifying the social world have had a considerable impact on the delivery of medicine and health care, promoting a standardization of practices. This is particularly so in relation to clinical practice.

The movement towards rationalization in public health, and the corresponding development of protocols, guidelines, decision support aides and various other instruments, encourage health practitioners, including primary care physicians and surgeons, to base clinical decisions on population health, and not simply the health of their individual patients. This is a fundamental change in clinical practice, as medical students have traditionally been trained to be patient advocates.

There has always been rationing of health services within clinical medicine, but this was largely implicit and the prerogative of the clinician. These instruments of rationalization represent a much more explicit form of rationing, the consequence of an insistence on efficiency. Here, public health decision makers and health service managers have seemingly acquired the capability to determine how the limited available resources are distributed so as to achieve the biggest overall health gain. Intrinsic to this utilitarian approach is the assumption that the inefficient use of health resources is unethical.

A drive for efficiency has not been the only means by which public health has impacted upon the work of health professionals. The emergence of risk factor epidemiology, which has been a major force in public health since the Second World War, has influenced the way health practitioners engage with patients. Health practitioners are tasked not only with diagnosing actual diseases, but also identifying which possible diseases a patient may be at risk of contracting, and subsequently intervening to reduce that risk. So alongside the health economist is another important colleague of the epidemiologist – the health promoter.

Risk factor epidemiology and health promotion have entered the clinic. Risk factor epidemiology arose out of efforts to explain and understand the main forces of mortality resulting from the epidemiological transition. No longer could germ theory hold sway as the dominant approach in public health: a multiple-cause theory of disease, particularly in relation to chronic diseases, has come to prominence. The emblematic event of risk factor epidemiology was the linking of lung cancer with smoking (Susser 1998). Consequently, this has encouraged a particular focus on the individual as the cause of future medical conditions. Risk factor epidemiology is particularly apt as a public health framework for the clinical consultation as it identifies factors in individuals that may make them susceptible to disease, in isolation from other individuals (with the exception of family who may share genetic predispositions). There is, within this framework, little regard for the social structures that shape individuals (ibid.). Just as the family physician or general practitioner can do little about class divisions in society, risk factor epidemiology elides the relationship between class divisions, or other social divisions, and illness and death.

Since it is primary health care physicians and general practitioners who are the health professionals most likely to have ongoing contact with members of the population, it is believed that they are well placed to persuade patients to adopt public health measures aimed at reducing the risk of a range of chronic diseases, particularly diabetes and heart disease. But this is not a simple task for health professionals. Complications do arise, and it is not always appropriate for primary care physicians and general practitioners to broach issues of preventive health with patients.

This chapter highlights another way in which public health extends its reach. It shows how a particular form of moral regulation that is developed in the sphere of public health is translated into another sphere – that of the clinical consultation. This chapter will outline some of the tensions that arise when public health infiltrates the clinical consultation and chart developments that resulted from the desire to promote economic efficiency in the provision of health services. It will then outline issues that clinicians face when public health interests in health promotion enter the clinic.

Standardizing Reforms

After the Second World War, there was optimism about the ability of health services to improve the health of the population vastly, and the health sector expanded significantly. By the 1970s, it became apparent that medicine could absorb resources indefinitely, and yet the returns were diminishing and major health problems remained (Marmor et al. 1994). As a result, there was a worldwide phenomenon of reining in health spending and the impact of health economics started to be felt. External challenges of ageing populations, technological developments in medicine, and changes in the macro-economy forced a re-examination of health delivery systems in an effort to provide more efficient and effective outcomes (Saltman 1994).

In the 1970s and 80s, ideas from economics started to make an impact on medicine, with medical journals developing an interest in notions like cost-effectiveness and marginal utility (Berg 1997). Traditionally, medicine as an institution has been relatively free from such external influences. It has been able to make strong arguments for determining how much money should be spent on health issues and why medical practitioners should be free to deal with problems as they see fit:

> Presenting itself as a 'science', medicine has been able to claim open-ended budgets on the strength of the alleged scientific link between needs and services provided. Presenting itself as a 'profession', medicine has been able to deflect any external examination of this relationship, retaining in the hands of the medical practitioners themselves responsibility for ensuring the linkage between medical care and health. (Lomas and Contandriopoulos 1994: 254)

Lomas and Contandriopoulos provide an illustrative example of the kind of argument that is made to standardize medical procedures. They argued that as the scientific basis of medicine has become questionable, there has been more willingness to question open-ended budgets and scrutinize the process of self-regulation. The challenge facing the public regulation of medicine is how to make the profession accountable for the quality of care and for the cost-effective use of resources (Lomas and Contandriopoulos 1994). To meet such a challenge, they argue that clinical epidemiological data on the relative worth of different interventions needs to be developed into guidelines for clinical practice, and monitoring and assessment of the individual and the profession needs to occur. There is an assumption here that the definitions of appropriate practice are neutral, as well as a tendency to valorize science as the arbiter of clinical decisions. Guidelines and protocols relate to efforts to standardize medicine, and as such to define medical practice as the logical and sequential application of science. These types of assumptions underlie the rationale of many health reforms in terms of calls for changes to clinical practice. The challenge to clinical autonomy through efforts to quantify clinical practice links with state calls for fiscal constraint, and together these form fundamental elements in health reforms internationally.

Disputes arose between those who called for cost constraints and rationing and those who felt this led to unmet needs. An anxiety over variability in clinical practice has further fostered attempts to standardize health service delivery, spawning a new sub-industry: 'variously labelled as quality assessment and assurance, continuous quality improvement, total quality management, managed care, utilization review, and outcomes research, all with roots either in clinical epidemiology or productivity enhancement' (Marmor et al. 1994: 226).

The move towards the standardization of clinical practice has, perhaps paradoxically, been facilitated by neo-liberalism. In the neo-liberal era efforts have been made in many nation-states to look to the market as a means of regulating human affairs. Widespread unease with rising costs and the quality of health care services has led to reforms in many countries. There has been reluctance, however, to leave health care completely open to market forces. A view that the market would fail to provide necessary health care to those who lack the capacity to participate as 'consumers' has led nation-states to retain ultimate control over health provision. Each country has dealt with this dilemma in its own idiosyncratic way, but this has generally involved a mix of government management, market-facilitated competition and health professional self-regulation. While it is hoped that this heavily regulated competition will go some way to addressing the problems of burgeoning health care costs, governments have sought to tackle high costs and variations in health service delivery by imposing standardized, uniform management systems on health providers. Consequently, health practitioners such as surgeons and primary care practitioners find themselves having to balance often intricate clinical interactions with the proscriptions of cost-focused funding agencies and the added pressures arising from competition.

Thomas Osborne's discussion of governmentality provides insight into the processes of contemporary health reforms and the movement towards simplification. There is, Osborne states, an essential indeterminacy in all government health policy. Government-funded health policy is often justified with the notion of 'the right to health'. For this notion to have any meaning, 'health' must be defined. But, as a biological or physiological concept, it falls 'outside of the direct remit of any health policy' (Osborne 1997: 179). Health cannot be a direct aspect of citizenship, but only an indirect one. At best, governments can only provide conditions that grant all citizens a roughly equal chance at acquiring health. Furthermore, 'health' lacks an absolute definition. What constitutes health tends to change as various forms of ill-health wax and wane. In the past, for example, health was characterized by an absence of various contagious diseases such as polio and diphtheria. Now that these are less prominent, health is conceived of in terms of having a low risk of cardiovascular disease, a particular body shape, and so on: 'each time government takes steps towards the target of "health", the thing itself escapes over the horizon' (ibid.: 180).

In the neo-liberal era, this indeterminacy is dealt with by defining health via a set of 'surrogate values' (Osborne 1997). These are goals and targets, set by the government, which enable the formation of a specific health policy, such as the implementation of prioritization criteria for particular treatments. Surrogate values, then, provide government policy with a 'health' that has some determinacy. One result of this is a series of measures which seek to operationalize health policy, such as audit measures and league tables (ibid.).

Economics and Clinical Autonomy

In achieving their impact on health care delivery, health economists have been highly critical of the health professions and policy makers. Alan Maynard, for example, strongly criticizes health care delivery in the U.K., noting that data on costs is poor, there is wide variation in clinical practice, there is little data on the effectiveness of particular services and what data there is tends to be ignored, and the majority of health care services have no proven scientific basis (Maynard 1995). In a utilitarian vein, Maynard argues that current health care delivery is an inefficient use of health resources and is therefore unethical as it deprives other patients of services. In order to combat this wasteful use of resources, health economists develop systems to quantify health outcomes so that costs can be effectively related to them (Ashmore et al. 1989; Seedhouse 1995). For Maynard, this quantification could be achieved by defining health as length and quality of life (Maynard 1996). In essence, the argument being put forward by proponents such as Maynard is that the clinical autonomy of medical practitioners undermines the efficient allocation of health resources (Maynard 1995). Measures are then needed to influence and monitor the behaviour of health practitioners.

In addition to quantifiable health indicators that can be the basis of audits and league tables, such as recovery rates, number of operations performed and length of waiting lists, health economists have developed the notion of 'quality adjusted life years' (QALYs). This refers to the 'life years' that a particular health care activity will produce and the quality of life the intervention will give, and these are then set against the cost of the activity. Those activities that give the most life years at high quality for the least cost will be prioritized. In order to determine QALYs, it is necessary to assess epidemiological research on the mortality and morbidity outcomes of disease processes, and on the impacts of interventions (obtained primarily through clinical trials), along with economic research on the estimated financial implications of various health procedures. These sorts of measures allow individual health and population health to become quantifiable, and facilitate a centralized authority to develop and impose standardized, uniform and rational health protocols. An impact of this process of standardization is an increasing insistence that clinicians consider health issues at a population level and not at an individual level – a change from being advocates for individual patients to guardians of the public good.

It is no surprise that the measures developed by health economists (what Osborne refers to as surrogate values) are attractive to those managing health care systems. They provide what decision makers would see as a relative simplicity, and they are in accordance with the rhetoric of cost-effectiveness and transparency. Subsequently, the medical profession has become subject to the standardizing stipulations of health funders, whether private or public.

A way to make sense of these reforms is to see them as part of a long historical process of simplification. James Scott argues that in high modernity, we witness a process whereby what was once socially 'messy' and opaque is rendered intelligible and legible and therefore conducive to administration. This process is achieved through rationalization and standardization. Scott gives the example of the measures necessary to promote various forms of statecraft, such as ensuring taxes could be collected, trade could occur efficiently, and military power could be enhanced. Measures have included imposing a standardized system of surnames to register populations, the construction of maps to identify property, and the standardization of weights and measures across regions so that trade could be undertaken with more surety (Scott 1998). Scott refers to the 'fiscal illegibility' of premodern times (ibid.: 39). With premodern forms of land use, an outsider would be unaware of how rights to land use were determined, as a complex array of considerations would come into play. For instance, some villagers might have rights at some time of the year and not other times, rights might change during a drought, and joint owners of land could not necessarily state that any specific part of the land was theirs. For state purposes of taxation and procurement of food, such a system was obviously very difficult to administer. To allow for fiscal legibility, local practices had to be changed so that individuals could be associated with particular plots of land. Tenure needed to be simplified, even if it did not reflect how people used the land.

We could consider, by analogy, a concept of 'clinical' legibility. Efforts over the last few decades have been made to overcome the diversity and variability of local clinical practices, to replace practical knowledge with formal systems – Quality Assurance (QA), Evidence-based Medicine (EBM), medical audits, priority settings and so on. The goal of such systems is to make the often messy and opaque clinical practices more quantifiable: they can be granted with 'value' and costed, and this therefore enables more centralized control over clinical activities. Processes of centralization are facilitated through this transformation of complex phenomena into objects of quantification (Porter 1995). Just as the fiscal illegibility of Scott's example is an outcome of variation in the local, contingent practice of those who own and work the land, clinical illegibility (from the point of view of those who wish to determine whether clinical resources are being used efficiently) is the consequence of the often complex and idiosyncratic interactions between clinicians and patients.

Theodore Porter (Porter 1995) makes evident that before clinical practice could be rendered legible and subject to standardized protocols, many other aspects had to be quantified. For example, doses of medication needed to be standardized. The biological assay to determine the potency of medications needed to be developed. In 1910 the cat unit for testing the potency of digitalis was mooted. A minimal fatal dose per kilogram of cat could be determined by feeding leaves to cats. Unfortunately cats were not standardized – so the process to render clinical experience legible required the standardization of experimental animals.

To accept the notion of a controlled clinical trial, the basis of EBM, would be to subordinate clinical judgements and medical ideas to the dominance of numbers. Claude Bernard, a famous nineteenth-century French advocate of experimental research, abhorred statistical inquiries: 'He wanted to examine the specific lesions and injuries to organs, not the average of many organs' (Hacking 1990: 71). Although attempts were made in the first half of the nineteenth century to assess the outcomes of some treatments by subjecting them to statistical tests, this was rejected as medicine was 'always concerned with the individual' and not 'facts without authenticity' (ibid.: 85). The use of statistical methods in medicine only began after 1900, and it was not until the 1940s that statistical tests gained a firm foothold in medical research, and not until 1946 that the first randomized controlled trial was undertaken when Austin Bradford Hill assessed the efficacy of streptomycin for the treatment of pulmonary tuberculosis (Porter 2006b).

The idea of comparing groups to look for statistically significant differences was a style of reasoning that was foreign and alien to nineteenth-century medical men. A great many more concepts needed to be accepted before clinical trials could become the norm. One important concept was the notion of 'normal' that could be compared with the deviant (Hacking 1990). Without a notion of a normal distribution of the population it was not possible to establish whether the responses one got from a therapeutic intervention were due to chance (therefore not outside the normal distribution) or due to some real effect (therefore 'deviating' in a positive way from a normal distribution). The notion of 'normal' that we use today, which is both a comparison with the pathological and an ideal that we strive for (as in norms of behaviour) did not take a hold on medical and social thought until the late nineteenth century. Once a notion of normal had been established, the deviant could be identified and the constraints around normality would become narrower and narrower.

The work of Scott, Porter and others suggests inexorable processes of standardization and rationalization in society, with medical practice, like other aspects of social life, being caught up in these processes. This same process of rationalizing and standardizing for the purposes of statecraft can be witnessed in the current shape of the clinical consultation, and public health or population health concerns are the vehicle by which such standardizing processes have occurred.

There are, however, problems with the imposition of standardization on a messy reality. As Scott suggests: 'Designed or planned social order is necessarily schematic; it always ignores essential features of any real, functioning social order' (Scott 1998: 6). Practical, local knowledge and informal, contingent processes are a necessary antidote to imposed, stifling simplification. This is seen in response to rationing in clinical decision-making, where practitioners develop their own informal systems. These informal systems allow practitioners to resist imposed, standardizing linear protocols while at the same time giving the appearance of adhering to protocol stipulations.

Setting Priorities and Limiting Variation

A common response to the increasing costs of the health care sector and a desire for efficiency has been to undertake 'priority setting' as a form of 'rationing'. Rationing describes 'the process by which resources are allocated to individuals at the point of service or programme delivery', and priority setting describes 'the process of determining the budgets, and their distribution, which constrain the decisions about who gets what' (Klein et al. 1996: 7). Prior to this effort to explicitly prioritize health services, health professionals themselves would decide who would receive what type of treatment. They did this within broadly defined categories with budget allocation decisions being made by politicians and managers (Cumming 1994). Although this allowed for flexibility, there were, as has been outlined, questions about the effectiveness and appropriateness of the services delivered by professionals (ibid.). Since the late 1990s, considerable effort has been made to move away from systems of implicit rationing to explicit rationing, where the rules of allocation are more transparent (Mechanic 1997). In order to make rationing transparent, criteria for prioritization such as need and ability to benefit have to be defined. To put this another way, those qualities that are legible to the economist, and quantifiable, become the basis for health rationing (Ashmore et al. 1989).

Nation-states have pursued a number of paths in attempting to achieve rationing of health services. Limits may be placed on the number of treatments that can be provided, as with the 'most draconian and thought-provoking' scheme devised in Oregon (Watts 2006). The Oregon Medicaid Initiative defined a basic package of health services that everyone could access (Birkmeyer and Welch 1993). Anything outside of that package was not paid for by the state and so people would either miss out or have to pay for the service out of their own pocket.

The debate over a core of health services or a basic package of services brought to the fore a number of issues that point to some of the tensions and contradictions within medicine. Firstly, it is assumed that medical practices are firmly entrenched in science. Yet the attack of health economists suggested that much of what is practised under the aegis of orthodox medicine has not had the sort of scientific validation that practitioners themselves might assume or expect. In the 1990s concerns were increasingly raised about the limited evidence for orthodox clinical practices. An editor of the *British Medical Journal* suggested that only about 15 per cent of medical interventions are supported by 'solid scientific evidence' (Smith 1991). This rhetoric provided a particular impetus for the EBM movement. Secondly, there is a constant tension between communal goals and individual goals. Who determines the 'morally defensible balance' between society and the individual (Haas 1994)? Should economists, accountants and managers make decisions based on explicit priorities, or should individual practitioners make judgements on medical and ethical grounds (Tenbensel 2000)? Should decisions be made by consensus or by some particular representatives?

In 1994 the Department of Health in Britain embraced the notion of knowledge-based medicine in which it was assumed that science could identify those treatments or procedures which were not effective, and from this resources could be freed up for those therapies identified as effective (Klein et al. 1996). Such measures aim to ensure that explicit criteria must be met before various services can be employed, that is, that only approved, cost-effective services and technologies are utilized and that there is some uniformity in terms of the services provided to various patients. In this tradition the National Institute for Health and Clinical Excellence (NICE) in Britain requires technology appraisals to recommend specific treatments (Steinbrook 2008).

Variability in treatment decisions, for example in primary care, was identified as a problem for several reasons. Variation suggests that some practitioners prescribe more drugs than others, or more expensive ones. Some practitioners may be referring patients on to other specialist services more often than others, and some may make greater use of laboratory services. Drugs, specialists and laboratory services are not cheap, and variations in the utilization of these courses of action suggest that practitioners are clearly not following the same protocols. Variation among clinicians also suggests that their activities are not firmly based in science: there must be other factors that influence, for instance, whether or not a patient will be referred to a specialist, that exacerbate variability. Policy developments have been enacted to overcome what has been seen as an inappropriate basis for rationing decisions, such as surgeon or patient lobbying (Dew et al. 2005a).

The variability of practice increasingly became a common worry in many countries from the 1990s and has had major implications for the medical profession. In their observation of events in Ontario, Canada, Coburn and colleagues cite examples of attempts to reduce variability in medical services that had been identified. In response to the Ministry of Health's perceived need to standardize practice, caps were placed on the spending of physicians and attempts were made to control the actual content of care. The Ministry of Health laid down explicit guidelines for medical practice (Coburn et al. 1997). Berg argues that terms like guidelines, protocols and practice policies have been used to describe the same thing, arguing that 'they can be read as a set of *instructions* telling medical personnel to do a certain thing in a certain situation' (Berg 1997: 2).

Quality assurance programmes and medical audits have become a common method to assist in achieving these aims of restricting health spending and limiting variation in service provision. This has not simply involved the subjection of practitioners and primary care givers to the dictates of government agencies or medical insurers, however. While political interests have driven the movement towards standardization and uniformity in health care, medical associations and practitioners themselves have taken a great deal of the responsibility for instigating the measures and regulating medical practice.

Ashmore and colleagues suggest that applying the methods of health economists 'will not mean that the irrationalities of political negotiation are being replaced by rational economic appraisal. It may mean that sections of management and various medical specialisms adopt the procedures and conclusions by economists and employ them selectively as a political resource' (Ashmore et al. 1989: 93).

One form of political negotiation attempting to make practitioners more accountable is through legislation that preserves the power of the medical profession as a whole by increasingly controlling individual practitioners. For example, in Ontario the state sought to deal with the burden of burgeoning health care costs by restricting individual practitioners, and the medical profession responded by attempting to put its own 'house in order' (Coburn et al. 1997). The state wishes to rationalize the delivery of medical services in order to control costs. For the state this is to ensure comparability allowing for the possible identification of areas where cost-savings can be made. For the medical profession, standardization is one element in ensuring the credibility of the profession in the eyes both of its funding agents and the public. Similarly, Freidson (1986) has observed that in the U.S., medical professions have responded to the movement towards accountability and cost-effectiveness by imposing their own restrictions on their practitioners, thus preserving a degree of power and autonomy for the profession as a whole. As Curtis and Taket (1996: 178) point out: 'In both the U.S.A. and the U.K., governments have accepted that medical audits should be carried out through peer review, which means that senior doctors, the most powerful actors in the health system, retain control over the process.' By having medical associations and peer-review systems govern individual practitioners, it is hoped that a degree of clinical freedom will be maintained while avoiding a large variation in services that can prevent the uniformity and predictability sought by health economists.

Various forms of quality assurance are now central components in the management of health care systems. As Jost defines it, in general terms quality assurance 'refers to programmes that set standards, assess the performance of professionals or institutions with respect to these standards, encourage improvement where performance can be improved, and attempt corrective action where the non-compliance is unacceptable' (Jost 1992: 70). While systems for checking, specifying and maintaining the quality of health care had been under development since the 1960s (Ellis and Whittington 1993), it was not until the 1980s that any explicit reference to quality assurance was made. Quality assurance programmes often involve medical audit studies which aim to identify problem areas within health care (maternal death rates, for instance) and develop ameliorative guidelines for practice. Individual practitioner medical audits, reviews of practitioners by colleagues or an external agent and the promotion of further education and training are also often part of these quality assurance programmes. Medical audit 'includes the analysis of procedures used for diagnosis and treatment, the use of resources and the resulting outcome and quality of life for the patient' (Rosenthal 1995: 136), and involves some attempt to provide 'objective criteria' for the management of clinical practice. Such objective criteria often arise from consensus conferences and an analysis of 'appropriate use of investigations and therapies' from which guidelines could be produced (ibid.: 137).

In England, developments in quality assurance were the result of a governmental push towards business management and a focus on efficiency, consumer service and accountability on the one hand, and the drive of the Royal Colleges to improve the practice of their clinicians on the other (Jost 1992). The British government confronted quality assurance issues directly in a 1989 Health Service White Paper produced by the Department of Health – *Working for Patients*. This paper proposed that compulsory medical audit programmes be established in both the hospital and primary care sector (Seale 1993). The British government, then, left it to the medical profession to establish its own audit procedures, though managers were tasked with the responsibility of ensuring that such procedures were implemented. The medical audit was mandated as a part of all doctors' contracts in the NHS. This method of providing quality assurance in clinical practice was also used in the U.S., where insurance companies also sought to limit the costs of medical care (ibid.).

While European medical professions still maintain a large element of control over the quality assurance programmes, practitioners in the U.S. are subject to more external controls. Such external controls include state physician licensure boards, and Medicare peer review organizations which are accountable to government. It is also not uncommon for U.S. judges and lay juries to assess the performance of doctors. Regulation in the U.S.A. also makes greater use of sanctions such as suspension of licenses and exclusion from federal health insurance programmes (Jost 1992).

Curtis and Taket suggest that quality control developments in the U.S. health sector indicate that there is 'a trend towards trying to monitor local variation in health service quality in terms of a limited range of quantifiable comparative indicators, available in a similar format for a large number of providers (Curtis and Taket 1996: 167). Indicators and quality measures include such things as immunization rates of children, prenatal care, and the management of illness. What we see in these moves is a compelling force towards the standardization of treatment in order to conform to the requirements of quality assurance committees. Calls for further integration of population-based and clinical approaches to address chronic health conditions, such as diabetes, are additionally likely to foster standardization processes (Fielding 2009).

Complex Clinical Practice and Resistance

There is resistance among practitioners and primary care givers to the rationalizing guidelines and protocols of policy makers, and resistance to adopting public health policy in clinical interactions. This is despite the fact that medical organizations have implemented and directed many of these measures themselves. There is a clash between measures to standardize practices and the interactions that take place during clinical practice: rationing procedures and stipulated protocols can interfere with clinical freedom, and many practitioners feel that it is the health of the patient that suffers as a result. Essentially, this clash is the consequence of a disjunction between the surrogate values used to define health employed by health economists, and the actual, far messier and complex realities of 'health' and 'illness' that clinicians must deal with.

Problems inherent in the use of QALYs illustrate this disjunction. One problem is the way decisions are made depending on how much value is assigned to life. If a human life is priced as being worth $1 million then decisions would be very different from pricing it at $200 million (Simmons and Scott 1998). The way we ration on the basis of QALYs may also go against our moral or ethical standards. We could ask, for example, if a donated kidney infected with hepatitis C should be used in renal transplantation. Using QALYs, it can be more efficient to use the infected kidney than to discard it (ibid.). QALYs have also been criticized for failing to measure quality of life that is unrelated to health. If we developed a system of rationing simply on the basis of QALYs, then people would not have access to services such as in vitro fertilization, for example. And in terms of providing health services, QALYs would place no value on information provided for its own sake (Devlin et al. 1999).

Criticisms have also been made of other measures, such as EBM, related to the rationing of health services. EBM aims to determine the most effective procedures on the basis of evidence from clinical trials. Once the effective procedures have been identified, guidelines for therapeutic treatment can be put in place.

The purported 'gold standard' of clinical trials is the double blind, placebo-controlled trial or the randomized controlled trial (RCT). If RCTs have not been, or cannot be carried out, then other forms of evidence are relied upon, including the consensus of 'experts'. So if controlled trials are not possible or have not been carried out then the vested interests of expert or consensus panels or other factors may come into play that influence recommendations made and the guidelines that are developed. However, there are also many problems with the gold standard of RCTs. Patients selected for controlled trials have tended to be middle-aged white males who have no coexisting conditions. This is based on the assumption that male physiology is less variable than female physiology, and therefore with males you are more likely to see the effect of the intervention. However, in clinical settings doctors are faced with a patient population that is far more diverse than this.

Furthermore, there is a difference between efficacy and effectiveness that bears upon the clinical use of EBM (Lohr et al. 1998). Efficacy requires that a clinical procedure achieve benefits to individuals in defined populations when it is applied under ideal circumstances. Effectiveness applies to the clinical setting, not a controlled setting, where a procedure should do more good than harm. Controlled trials tend to test for efficacy and not effectiveness. Many interventions found by RCT to be efficacious do not lead to improved outcomes when translated into practice (Glasgow et al. 1999). This is exacerbated by the increasing tendency to conduct RCTs for pharmaceuticals in what are termed 'non-traditional' research areas (for example, Latin America and Eastern Europe) by commercial companies (Petryna 2007). Petryna reports a scientific advisor of a contract research organization stating that 'companies can now pick and choose populations in order to get a most pronounced drug benefit signal as well as a "no-harm" signal'. This is achieved through trial recruitment strategies, which, for example, can recruit from 'treatment-naive' groups who have very little history of pharmaceutical use, but the results are generalized to 'treatment-saturated' markets with many people on multiple medications (ibid.).

In addition, there is something besides science that is being used in clinical assessments: the 'experiential knowledge of the medical profession' (Klein et al. 1996: 104). 'Effectiveness' and 'outcomes' represent values, and not scientific universals. Outcomes may be seen as good from the doctor's perspective, but not necessarily from the patient's, and so on (ibid.). Calculations regarding effectiveness are based on groups, and different conclusions may be drawn when we consider individual patients, where the benefits of a particular intervention may be greater. Furthermore, some technologies may be ineffective when first developed, and thus score poorly, even though modifications would result in improvement. In this light, it can be concluded, 'Neither science nor economics will resolve the pain of choice' (ibid.: 139).

Similarly, for many surgical specialities, the evidence to support decision making is not available, and even where validity studies of prioritization tools have been undertaken, the relationship between these studies and clinical practice has not been established (Conner-Spady et al. 2004). Protocols and standardization measures, then, are highly problematic for those working with patients and are often resisted in a number of ways. Many practitioners feel that protocols conflict with clinical autonomy: they lack flexibility, and this has been one reason for the limited acceptance of rationing processes by surgeons (McLeod et al. 2004). Rationing criteria are perceived as not reflecting clinical judgement (ibid.).

Clinical standardizing tools can be used in a variety of ways when introduced. For example, tools developed to determine whether someone should have access to elective surgery in the public hospital system in the Otago region of New Zealand include such criteria as social functioning and patient characteristics. Social functioning is assessed in terms of 'the ability to care for self or others, or to work, or in terms of other economic/lifestyle impacts' and patient characteristics include the patient's attitude to surgery.[1] Clinicians have to assign a value to these criteria. When filling out such tools, clinicians may game scores by adding more points than is warranted to ensure that their patients are prioritized, or they may weight subjective criteria differently. If they game then other patients in the region who have greater need may miss out on treatment. Awareness of such an outcome can promote clinicians to think of health outcomes at a population level, instead of advocating for the particular patient they are dealing with (Dew et al. 2005a). However, the different weighting that clinicians might give to the same criterion works against the goal of overcoming variability, and also lacks transparency. So, even when protocols and guidelines are developed, a certain level of clinical autonomy is maintained and rationing can remain implicit.

The view that we act on the basis of pre-specified plans has been critiqued, in part on the basis that any rules can be rendered inappropriate as a result of the specific circumstances that they confront (Heath and Luff 2000). The immediate context of action, in this case decision making, can undermine the application of the rule, and resolution is found in the commonsense reasoning of individuals and the real-time actions of others. The consultation is an 'ongoing collaborative accomplishment' of activities (ibid.: 21).

In a footnote to her discussion of Erving Goffman, Rawls argues that 'informalities are an inescapable part of any organization, and that attempts to eradicate them simply multiply informal practices' (Rawls 1990: 80). A breach of the rules of institutional norms has quite different consequences from the breach of rules of what Rawls terms the Interaction Order Sui Generis. The interaction order involves rules of everyday interaction that are based on moral obligations of reciprocity. To breach these rules has immediate effects for selfhood in terms of embarrassment, shame and so forth. To breach institutional rules has no such immediate sanction. Hence, as is seen when actual consultations between surgeons and patients are examined, surgeons work hard to maintain the Interaction Order of the consultation. However, they may set aside, or not have explicit regard to, attempts to impose institutional norms of prioritization that do not clearly relate to the requirements of the Interaction Order (Dew et al. 2010). Obligations to the actual interaction override obligations to impersonal documents.

The following illustrates the interactional delicacy required to gain a patient's consent to go forward with further diagnostic procedures (taken from Dew et al. 2010). The context here is that Patient A has undergone some investigative procedures after being ill, and has returned to consult her surgeon. Patient A is happy in her belief that she now experiences good health. The surgeon begins with an enquiry to find out from the patient what her perspective is in relation to her health, asking her how she is. She responds with 'good'. The surgeon points out that she has an obstruction of the bowel, to which the patient replies that indeed she was 'very fluorescent yellow' for three months, but is obviously not so now. The surgeon then asks how her general health had been prior to that, and again the response is 'good'.

The surgeon continues to try to find a way to change the patient's optimistic belief about her health status and deliver some bad news in a delicate manner. And so this pattern of asking about aspects of her health and getting a positive response is repeated nine times in the consultation. The surgeon breaks this cycle finally by asking if doctors had explained that a blockage such as hers in the bile duct is 'normally' a growth and that you have to assume that it is a malignancy, which then requires checking out. But by this time the patient has augured that bad news is on the way, and is now not only prepared to alter her optimism about her present condition, but suggests the way forward in terms of getting further investigations. The point of dwelling on this kind of example is that it indicates that following a checklist that adds up to a particular score that then determines what is to be done is inappropriate in many circumstances. The surgeon had to undertake a great deal of interactional work to get the patient to align with the required path of action. Any paperwork required to 'prioritize' the patient can be completed after such an interaction rather than determine the outcome of the interaction, as would be the required procedure if the goal of reducing variability and standardizing decision making is to be achieved.

So protocols can also be used after clinical decisions have already been made. The previous example illustrates this in a difficult case where there is a need for follow-up investigations. The following interaction relates to a consultation about eye surgery (Dew et al. 2010). The patient concerned needs the surgery and the consultant can get the surgery done. But what we see is an extra process added, whereby a nurse comes in after the consultation to administer a tool to determine how much the impairment is impacting on the patient's life, which is meant to determine whether the patient receives surgery or not.

The pro forma process of getting a nursing assessment done for 'accountability' purposes is seen when the consultant ends the consultation with: 'we just need to do some paper work now'. When the nurse comes in to do the scoring she opens with: 'okay let's do this quick and then you can get out of here'. Needless to say the score came out high enough so that the consultant could go ahead and arrange the surgery. But this illustrates a process whereby the form is filled out to match the decision and not the other way around.

Researchers have suggested that patients also 'misuse' the standardization systems. Particular patients were more able to 'work the system' to obtain care earlier than others. Consequently, it is not clear whether those patients getting care are those that necessarily have the greatest need (Bloomfield et al. 1999). In such cases the notion of equitable treatment, a basic goal of public health, is undermined.

QALYs, EBM, and priority-setting measures, then, can in practice be poor methods for determining health care provision. This point can be demonstrated by looking at the clinical interaction as a complex 'interactional achievement'. A bureaucratic model of clinical decision making will utilize knowledge-based algorithms to determine who should get treated and how, and will lay down formal rules of conduct for practitioners. But in so doing 'it undermines the flexible discretionary judgement that is necessary to adapt services to individual needs' (Freidson 1994: 193). Furthermore, the complex work of the doctor–patient consultation may not necessarily be 'rational' in terms of a purely linear bureaucratic logic (Dew et al. 2010). The consultation may involve the breaking of bad news, or ensuring that the views of the participants align so that there is no conflict over the treatment plans. Surgeons can carefully gauge a patient's reaction to talk of possible surgery without having to explicitly ask if the patient wants the surgery. The surgeon works, interactively, to ensure that he or she is aligned with the patient's view on how to proceed (ibid.). Following a protocol circumvents this interactional achievement and is likely to undermine it. A clinical consultation is more than the delivery of a service: it is an interactional accomplishment.

The interactional work involved in the delivery of diagnosis and medical assessment facilitates patient cooperation and commitment to professional understandings (Heath 1992). The use of protocols to promote efficiency and population-based benefit may be a blunt instrument, which potentially undermines the delicate and intricate work undertaken in consultations.

Public Health in the Clinic

As noted, there has been a movement encouraging practitioners to adopt a public health advocacy orientation when dealing with individual patients. Health promotion talk and risk epidemiology talk in the clinical consultation can be labelled 'lifestyle talk'. The WHO, for example, has implemented lifestyle interventions in primary care (McAvoy et al. 1999). In many countries, patients themselves are likely to include lifestyle talk in consultations, a result in part of public health promotions of healthy lifestyle (Hansen and Easthope 2007). Governments have endorsed the role of health professionals in providing lifestyle advice in order to help combat such conditions as heart disease and cancer. The U.K. government, in its *Our Healthier Nation* report, identified healthy living advice as a key component of its strategy (McAvoy et al. 1999). Consequently, health promotion is now regarded as a key component of clinical practice (McAvoy 2000) and health professionals are regarded as being well placed to influence patients wanting to quit smoking and to intervene to reduce alcohol consumption (Gray 2007). Other health promotion activities include screening, lifestyle counselling and 'well health' checks (McKinlay et al. 2005). Primary care initiatives to encourage changes in lifestyle include 'Green Prescriptions' where general practitioners and nurses prescribe exercise, which involves support for such things at attending fitness programmes.

The tension between the clinical encounter and public health promotion also relates to the interactional complexity of the practitioner's work. This tension is nicely demonstrated in the words of Beatrice Webb who campaigned for universal health care systems in the late nineteenth and early twentieth century. She was wary of the role that doctors in private practice play in undermining public health messages. As she argued, any doctor:

> dependent for a livelihood on a wide popularity among his ignorant patients, cannot be expected to run counter to their prejudices and to offer them, instead of the 'bottle of physic', stern advice as to the need for physical control, and as to the fatal effects of not altering their careless or intemperate habits of life. Where the patient chooses the doctor, he chooses the doctor whose methods and manners he likes best, not the one most likely to prevent the recurrence of the disease. (Cited in Sturdy 2002a: 247–48)

Primary care practitioners, whether in a fee-for-service situation or not, are faced with a particular dilemma when it comes to health promotion in the clinical consultation.

Lifestyle advice can be viewed as victim-blaming (Lawlor et al. 2000). Many health promotion activities touch on delicate topics and practitioners find themselves having to avoid causing emotional distress; suggesting that a patient should lose weight invokes the stigma of obesity and often involves enquiries into private activities of consumption and physical activity. Similarly, addressing a patient's alcohol or tobacco intake may be taken to imply deficits of self-control. Many practitioners feel that delving into particularly sensitive issues such as these is unnecessary, particularly when the patient's reason for being at the consultation is an unrelated issue. Also, lifestyle advice could be depicted as interfering with the way people choose to live, and in this, potentially disrupting the doctor–patient relationship (ibid.).

Many primary care physicians are ambivalent about the impact that lifestyle talk has on patients. As a consequence, it is felt that such a focus is not a good use of time within the context of time-pressured consultations (McKinlay et al. 2005). Some practitioners are, indeed, actively hostile to the idea of preventive medicine in clinical practice, suggesting that it is 'aggressively assertive, pursuing symptomless individuals and telling them what they must do to remain healthy' (Sackett 2002). Disasters in preventive medicine can be cited, such as the advice for postmenopausal women to take estrogen and progestin to protect against cardiovascular disease. This was poor advice, as the opposite effect was achieved (ibid.). So although it has been argued that general practitioners and primary care physicians are ideally suited to health promotion activities due to the frequent contact they have with the majority of the population (McAvoy et al. 1999), the actual practice of health promotion is by no means overwhelmingly endorsed by clinicians.

In Finland, for example, alcohol consumption is seen as a delicate topic that practitioners are reluctant to engage in (Aira et al. 2003; Lindfors and Raevaara 2005). To deal with this delicacy, doctors do not usually ask questions about alcohol at the beginning of any lifestyle talk, but discuss other issues first – such as diet, exercise and smoking, and as such the alcohol consumption question is subsequently able to be presented in a 'neutral' manner (Lindfors and Raevaara 2005). This does not apply to all questions regarding lifestyle however. New Zealand data shows that when GPs simply ask a patient if they smoke, patients who do often respond by discussing how they have tried or will try to give up (Major, n.d.). This could be read as patients being immediately defensive about a habit that has been successfully demonized through public health research and interventions.

Lifestyle talk also shows evidence of intriguing gender differences. Finnish research has shown that GPs respond differently to male and female patients in regard to the topic of alcohol consumption. When men state how much alcohol they consume, GPs then ask them to specify how much they drink. Women, however, proffer this information without being prompted (Lindfors and Raevaara 2005). Men will talk about 'non-problem' drinking by alluding to only drinking in their free time on evenings and weekends, and not every day, whereas women refer to drinking in company and at parties (ibid.). Patients, then, appear to be referencing particular, gender-specific norms of drinking: for men drinking is to be expected and does not need to be explained, but for women this is not the case.

Erving Goffman's work on the concept of 'face' provides a useful way to make sense of these tensions in the clinic. Goffman, influenced by Durkheim's work on social solidarity, developed the concept of face based on the assumption that morality is not something that is imposed upon us, but is rather something that is desired and desirable (Goffman 2006). Face is 'the positive social value a person effectively claims for himself by the line others assume he has taken during a particular contact' (Manning 1992: 38). In order for social situations to be saved – or some form of social order to be maintained – all parties must work to save their own face and save the face of others. As such, face maintenance is a condition of social interaction – social interaction itself cannot be maintained without considerations of face. To maintain face, participants in an interaction monitor each other and routinely combine together to sustain each other's dignity.

Topics related to lifestyle can be face-threatening in many ways. The common public health related issues of alcohol, smoking and diet can all potentially stigmatize the patient. Any lifestyle habits that are outside of a prescribed norm can be seen as 'character blemishes', and as such bring discredit on the specific person (Goffman 1963). Bringing attention to these character blemishes, while seeking to maintain the social interaction and the face of the participants, is understandably a challenging task.

Discussion

Risk factor epidemiology and the application of economics can be seen as part of a quantification rhetoric. As Petersen and Lupton argue, 'quantification rhetoric tends to suggest the figures used are not subject to doubt or uncertainty' (Petersen and Lupton 1996: 38). The concept of quantification rhetoric suggests that the power of quantification is not that it indicates an objective measurement of some aspect of the real world, but that turning aspects of the real world into numbers provides a sense of certainty that has a particularly persuasive power.

It has been argued here that recent decades have seen the assemblage of an extremely powerful standardization apparatus in health care. This apparatus combines quantification rhetoric with, amongst other things, management systems that bring together computer technologies and the use of protocols, health economics and rationing, population health perspectives and a particular scientific hierarchy that valorizes the randomized controlled trial as a source of authority.

Managerial approaches have been increasingly related to public health approaches, where there is a shift from clinical advocacy for particular patients to a population perspective with a focus on the best use of limited resources. In addition, health strategies have sought to encourage primary health care physicians to adopt public health measures, particularly in relation to smoking, nutrition, and physical activity. As such, public health can be seen to 'get right inside' the clinical encounter.

The increasing expectation that doctors will engage in lifestyle talk brings public health into the confined spaces of consulting rooms in face-to-face interaction. This is something quite different from public health campaigns that focus on advertising and education to whole groupings or even the entire population. Not only does risk factor epidemiology place constraints on the clinical autonomy of practitioners in terms of underpinning medical audits and quality assurance, but it also poses particular difficulties for the doctor–patient relationship.

There has been a shift from 'indeterminate expert-based medical autonomy toward technical evidence-based medical accountability' (Rappolt 1997: 977). The development of accountability and assurance mechanisms in health policy is not simply driven by the economic concerns of government. With therapies now increasingly required to be justified before a distrustful public, 'the appeal to impersonal rules became a very effective tool in the adjudication of medical uncertainty' (Matthews 1995: 146). The defence that the physician was the only one who could recognize the idiosyncrasies of the individual patient and administer therapies unique to that patient lost ground.

However, there are forms of resistance to these seemingly inexorable forces of rationalization and standardization in the clinic. Clinicians can undermine, sometimes through necessity, the attempts to simplify and make accountable their actions. Goffman's concept of face-work provides some insight into this process. Drawing on Durkheim, it can be argued that the moral forces that promote social solidarity concurrently provide some restraint on rationalization processes.

Notes

1. This Clinical Priority Assessment Criteria (CPAC) tool was accessed at www.cdhb.govt.nz/documents/VAS-CPAC-tool-May-07.pdf on 7 May 2010.

CHAPTER 5
The Political Use of Public Health

Introduction

Exposure to hazards in any setting can give rise to disputes over the impact of those exposures. U.S. Vietnam War veterans in America alleged that they suffered various symptoms due to exposure to Agent Orange, a herbicide that contained, as a by-product, dioxin (Scott 1988). Dioxin is perhaps the most toxic agent produced during chemical manufacture and in the event of dioxin contamination a host of symptoms can occur, including severe skin rashes, malaise, peripheral nervous system disturbances, liver toxicity and possibly cancer (Commission for the Environment 1985). In the process of attempting to gain recognition for their suffering, the Vietnam veterans ('Vets') were involved in disputes over the amount and type of exposure, whether the symptoms were uniquely associated with exposure or not, the effects of exposure on humans, and the time lag between exposure and consequence. Public health researchers, epidemiologists and occupational physicians are central in such disputes and frequently play a role in denying claims from those, like the Vets, who link their suffering to hazard exposure.

What we see in many disputes of this nature is an acceptance of the null hypothesis as the appropriate way to dismiss any possible consequences of exposure to hazardous substances or situations. In the null hypothesis of the scientific tradition the proposition is that the effect under consideration is not produced by the suspected cause (Scott 1988). Thus the greater sin, so to speak, is to implicate a causal mechanism when there is not one, than to miss the causal connection. In other words, in determining cause there is an overwhelming scientific desire to avoid false positives (where we determine that something is the cause when it is not), but a willingness to accept false negatives (where we determine that something is not the cause when it is). This is at the very heart of the political use of public health: vested interests can draw on 'good' scientific practices of public health researchers and scientists to support their efforts to dismiss claims against them.

Public health practice is informed by an epidemiological picture of population health and the distribution of disease. Yet, a glance through the popular press will indicate that epidemiological studies can come up with conflicting results (Watterson 1994). One day you may read that alcohol is bad for you, another day that red wine is good. Similarly, there have been debates over such issues as whether screening men for prostate cancer is a good use of resources, and whether or not mammography screening should be freely available for women under the age of fifty. Like all specialized sciences, experts are commonly engaged in debates about what constitutes knowledge, and what is the best way to utilize such knowledge. As ongoing arguments such as these illustrate, it is impossible to be absolutely certain about the findings of science.

Conflicts do not only occur amongst academically trained epidemiologists. Lay people often become involved in conflicts. A particular group in the community may become so concerned about an issue that they conduct their own research, producing findings that contest the views of trained experts. In the latter part of the twentieth century, there was an emergence of national environmental justice movements, particularly in the U.S., including the People of Color Environmental Movement and the Anti-Toxics Movement. These movements have adopted aspects of public health models of illness prevention to make sense of the threat of environmental harm and its effects on the population, and to identify those responsible for pollution (Brulle and Pellow 2006). This has been called lay or popular epidemiology (Brown 1989). These social movements often challenge experts on the causes and determinants of an illness. A celebrated example of popular epidemiology occurred in Woburn, Massachusetts, where local residents noted that a number of children in their area had contracted leukaemia. Residents traced the cause of this to the leaching of industrial waste into their water supply, and then successfully took the firms responsible to court (ibid.). This later became the basis for the film *A Civil Action*, starring John Travolta. Cases such as this are not uncommon, and as this chapter will illustrate, public health experts are often embroiled in these disputes.

Ulrich Beck draws a dramatic parallel between the public's response to environmental degradation and animal experimentation: 'A permanent experiment is being conducted … in which people serving as laboratory animals in a self-help movement have to collect and report data on their own toxic symptoms *against* the experts sitting there with their deeply furrowed brows' (Beck 1992: 69). Popular epidemiology can be seen as a response to the limitations of public health. Public health officials and epidemiologists work within a specific framework, what could be called a scientific-political framework, which compels them to adopt a particular stance when disputes over the possible cause of an illness arise. This is a stance that demands a very high standard of proof. To establish such proof, the hurdles faced by the U.S. war veterans, as well as a host of other hurdles, have to be negotiated. This can be contrasted with another possible stance, a 'balance of probabilities' stance, where evidence is weighed up to discern the most probable case.

Similar dichotomous positions can relate to the production of new hazards. We could deploy a high standard of proof, that any new substance or new process has to be shown to cause damage to people and the environment if we are to stop the substance from being released or new processes from being deployed. Or we could use the 'precautionary principle'. According to the Rio Declaration on Environment and Development, the precautionary principle is to be applied to conditions where there are threats of serious damage and there is a lack of scientific certainty. In such a situation, a course of action should be decided upon that assumes the worst-case scenario (Grey et al. 2007). The precautionary principle, however, is seldom invoked. In the example of toxic waste contamination, epidemiological evidence can be used to generate hypotheses, but it is rarely able to provide answers, and consequently no course of action can be decided upon (ibid.). As Ulrich Beck has illustrated, it is difficult to restrain activities that may have seriously deleterious effects when no solid answers can be provided. Public health researchers and scientists are often pivotal in this provision of scientific data that offers no answers.

Science expertise, then, is often used to reify a stance requiring a high standard of proof before ameliorative action can be taken. When a community group becomes concerned about an issue, and the burden of proof is too high and difficult to attain, a social movement can develop that pitches lay people and their popular epidemiology against the claims of public health expertise, and those of the parties with vested interests: usually either government or business. The public's trust in public health officials can be undermined as a result. By way of illustration, in the Love Canal scandal in New York State, where residential housing was built on a toxic waste site, many in the local community concluded that the 'Departments of public health have become departments of public reassurance' (Ozonoff and Boden 1987). These sorts of challenges to public health are symptomatic of an era characterized by a concern with the environment, pollution and the management of risk, and where trust in experts has become eroded.

This chapter will begin with a discussion of what the sociologist Ulrich Beck has referred to as the risk society. The intensification of industrial production and technology has brought about potentially catastrophic hazards that have the capacity to affect all members of society. We are also, as Anthony Giddens points out, heavily reliant on experts. The systems we have developed to support our lives are so complex that we depend upon specialists to provide advice on how best to manage ourselves in relation to these systems. This has led to a tension between experts and officials on the one hand, and the public on the other (Giddens 1991). This chapter will go on to illustrate specific examples of this tension, highlighting how public health experts can overlook the complexities of working and living with hazards, thus perpetuating risk. We will also see instances of how disputes are settled, and the inability of science to provide certainty. This uncertainty can be used by various interests to avoid accountability – public health scientists' claim to science, but public health scientists' inability to provide certainty, is central to what Ulrich Beck terms 'organized irresponsibility'. In short, the chapter explores the conflict between public health as a science deploying the standard methodologies of science, and public health as an agent of social justice. By deploying the very standards of science, public health can work against its concern for social justice. Durkheim identified this sort of tension in his cult of humanity, which had to be based on science, but also went beyond science.

Risk and the Erosion of Trust

Ulrich Beck argues that we have moved from modernity to an age of reflexive modernity. As he suggests, reflexive modernity is characterized by 'societies that are confronted by the challenge of the self-created possibility, hidden at first, then increasingly apparent, of the self-destruction of all life on this earth' (Beck 1995: 67). Aside from producing needed goods, the forces of production have always generated public harms: environmental dangers and pollution. Industrial production has spread and become embedded throughout the world, and as a result these side effects have become rife. Consequently, risk has emerged as 'a central cultural construct in the twentieth century' and 'our cultural and political responses to it, the ways we define, assess and symbolise the risks it is seen to pose – are central, not marginal, to an understanding of the social world in which we live' (Phillimore and Moffatt 1999: 139).

The contemporary world is fraught with risks brought about by widespread technological changes. There are of course numerous hazards faced, such as those resulting from the production of chemicals, nuclear power, the use of pesticides, insecticides and herbicides, and more recent developments in genetic engineering and nanotechnology. Beck argues that there are several key characteristics that make this 'risk society' distinct from previous societies. Firstly, in contemporary risk society hazards affect all social classes. In the past, exposure to hazards was more common for those who lacked wealth, whereas today, hazards encompass a geographical and spatial totality (Beck 1995). Because the productive forces of industrial societies have become so effective at delivering needed goods, there has been a shift in focus away from the 'need' to produce goods towards a 'concern for the risks' of producing such goods (Barnes 1995). Unlike concerns around poverty, where there are insufficient goods for the poor, this anxiety over public harms can affect everyone: 'poverty is hierarchic, smog is democratic' (ibid.: 107).

Second, the rules of causality and guilt have eroded. This is due to the difficulty of gaining proof that an identified problem is caused by a particular technology; the burden of proof in identifying a particular agent as causal is extremely one-sided, disadvantaging those who have misgivings about the technology in question (Beck 1995). We see this playing out in the specific case of the Vietnam War veterans. Because of this, there tends to be an increase in hazards, as those resisting the introduction and use of hazardous technologies find the burden of proof an insurmountable obstacle. Beck suggests:

> The injured parties, i.e. (almost) everybody, can never complete the obstacle race of impossibilities. First, they must demonstrate the injury; second, they must give proof that a given substance was indeed what gave rise to the injury; third, they must prove

> that the substance originates in a named company; and, fourth, they must finally accomplish the task, impossible against the inertial mass of data, of suing one person for legal responsibility. (Beck 1995: 131)

The prevalence of dangers worldwide adds to the difficulty of proving that a single substance is the cause of any particular problem (ibid.).

A third characteristic of risk society is that hazards may be minimized, but can never be eliminated. Safety guarantees may be imposed and tightened, but are, in reality, no guarantee. Risk, then, is unavoidable. Finally, there is a lack of provision for catastrophe. Large-scale hazards (nuclear, chemical, industrial) can potentially cause irreversible damage with no foreseeable end, and no possible economic compensation could ameliorate such damage. Beck uses the example of the Chernobyl catastrophe to illustrate some of the inherent contradictions of risk society. In April 1986 Unit Number Four of the nuclear power plant in Chernobyl, in the Ukraine, exploded, causing the world's worst nuclear disaster and sending a radioactive cloud across Europe (Holt 2010). Despite the possibility that a meltdown at a nuclear power station could occur, no preparations for dealing with such an event were made in advance. People in Germany, 2,000 km away from Chernobyl, were told that there was no hazard to their health; yet at the same time they were instructed to avoid being out in the rain, avoid walking on their lawns, and shower their children after having been outside.

Unsurprisingly, given the Chernobyl catastrophe and the response to it, reflexive modernity is also characterized by a loss of faith in science. In the past, science has been employed to determine and understand 'risks', whereas the population simply perceived risk. In other words, science enjoyed a monopoly over defining 'hazards', while the public were positioned as prone to irrational and unscientific perceptions (Beck 1992). In contemporary times this distinction is no longer tenable. Unlike the dogmas of religion and tradition, Beck explains, the dogmas of science have within them the standards of their own critique (ibid.). In effect, the knowledge produced by science fails to meet its own strict criteria for certainty. As a result, scientific scepticism will increasingly be applied to science itself, and 'scientific civilization is subjecting itself to a publicly transmitted criticism that shakes its foundations and its own self-conception' (ibid.: 156). Furthermore, science can exacerbate the generation of risk. When science is used to determine the acceptable levels of use, for instance, of a potentially hazardous herbicide, it legitimates its use, resulting in the further dissemination of risk (ibid.). In his polemical fashion, Beck states that scientists provide a blank cheque to poison nature.

A number of criticisms have been levelled at Beck. His view that risk has replaced need seems a peculiar one when taken in the context of poverty and food shortages in many parts of the world. What is perceived to be a risk is then context-dependent. He has also been criticized for overemphasizing differences in the experience of risk in premodern times (Elliott 2002). His argument that class is not a central feature of reflexive modernity has been argued against as, for example, it ignores the persistence of socio-economic inequalities (Atkinson 2007). At a theoretical level Beck has been accused of drawing on rational-choice and utilitarian understandings of risk (Elliott 2002). In addition Beck's solution to the problems of reflexive modernity pivot around new forms of self-control and self-limitation, to which he argues there are no constraints. Others argue that the view that risk production is controllable remains a 'chimera' (Smart 1996). Nevertheless, Beck's argument brings into focus the salience of risk and the impact of human action in the production of hazards in contemporary society.

Anthony Giddens makes a similar characterization of contemporary times. Giddens (1991) argues that 'manufactured uncertainty' and 'manufactured risk' are central elements of contemporary society. These have their origin in the prevalence of science, technology and industry which, in effect, 'disembed' social relations from the contexts of action. That is, important relationships are increasingly with people at a distance, or who are anonymous. Due to the complexity of the many systems that we have created to aid and assist our lives, individuals cannot possibly understand or control all the forces that affect them. These systems have extended into areas of life previously governed by traditional forms of social organization (Higgs and Jones 2001). In other words, we have to invest a great deal of trust in vicarious relationships with a vast range of people, which could include landlords, those who design public transport systems, airline pilots, bureaucrats in government departments, and so on.

Thus, the character of trust in contemporary times is not so much related to known individuals, but relates to a faith in the workings of systems and processes in situations where one possesses limited knowledge (Giddens 1991). Personal trust, then, is being replaced by impersonal trust, and there is a heavy reliance on the experts of various specialized fields.

In premodern cultures, kinship provided a stabilizing network that endured across time and space. Localized relations organized in terms of place afforded familiarity, consistency and therefore trust. In addition, the moral interpretations of life supplied by religion imparted a sense of security. An emphasis on tradition provided for routines that connected the present with the past and the future. Risk in premodern cultures revolved around threats from nature, such as infectious diseases and natural disasters, threats from human violence as a result of marauding armies, and a threat posed by a fall from religious grace. On the other hand, in a disembedded modern society, Giddens argues that threats are a result of what he terms reflexive modernity, human-made threats such as climate change and environmental degradation. Threats are a result of our own activities (Giddens 1990).

Security, for Giddens, rests upon a balance of trust and acceptable risk. In relation to science there is ambivalence in this relationship between trust and risk. Trust is a necessary result of the incapacity to be fully informed about science and technology, but there also exists scepticism about the claims to specialist knowledge of scientific experts. As such, trust in experts is fragile. Giddens suggests that in fact there is a constant tension between experts and officials on the one hand, and lay actors on the other, over the appropriation of knowledge (Giddens 1991).

Irwin and colleagues demonstrate in their case study of residential areas sited close to chemical factories that the public have high levels of mistrust of technical and scientific sources where there may be commercial interests involved (Irwin et al. 1996). Similarly, Wynne shows the mistrust of state interests in the case of nuclear power in Britain (Wynne 1996).

Both Beck and Giddens present a scenario in which science and industry have created a world where risk is widespread, the hazards we face are potentially catastrophic, and the authority of science is being undermined. Experts have been entrusted to manage the various complex systems of modern living, but tension is common between these experts and lay people. These are the conditions under which public health experts operate. Medicine and health represent complex, highly specialized areas of knowledge and practice, and the public has entrusted various experts (practitioners, public health officials, epidemiologists, and so on) to oversee medical systems, recommend interventions and provide advice on healthy and safe living.

Determining Risk and Creating Hazards

Public health officials are often involved in determining acceptable, safe levels of exposure to hazardous substances, and providing protocols for those who must work with such substances. These protocols, however, can be highly problematic: they are developed using simplified models that may have little in common with the complexities encountered by those who must interact with hazardous substances, either in the work place or in other settings. So, just as we saw in chapter 4 that protocols do not match the interactional complexities of consultations, here workplace protocols on the handling of hazardous substances do not match the circumstances of actual work practices.

Brian Wynne has explored disparities between the standardized risk assessment and the actual risk encountered when hazardous substances are used, which nicely illustrates the gap between expert and lay knowledge of risk. In the 1970s in the U.K., a government agency concluded that the pesticide 2,4,5-T was safe for public use, yet the experience of agricultural workers using the pesticide led them to lobby for a reinvestigation. The Committee on the safety of pesticides asserted that the pesticides safety was conditional upon its proper manufacture, distribution and use; a set of stipulations that the committee assumed were unproblematic. For the workers, it was the very conditions in which the pesticide was used that raised concerns (Wynne 1987). First of all, drums of 2,4,5-T often arrived defaced or with no labels describing proper conditions of use. Secondly, the organizational realities of farm labour meant that workers could not refuse to spray because the weather conditions were wrong or because the protective equipment was defective or non-existent. Thirdly, additives were used to speed-up the action of the spray, despite the effects of this being unknown. Fourthly, new spraying technologies were developed which could potentially give rise to greater exposure by producing, for instance, a finer spray. Also the culture of the workplace did not encourage workers to fear or be mindful of risk.

Thus, there was a considerable disparity between the ideal working conditions assumed by the experts and the actual reality of the workers. As a result, exposures to hazardous conditions were not able to be avoided, as the experts had assumed. Wynne's analysis alerts us to the ways in which experts exclude the reality of a situation in their assessment of risk, where lay accounts of risky activities are usually seen as irrational or anecdotal in nature and tend to be ignored.

Wynne also discusses the responses of Cumbrian hill farmers in the English Lake District to the expert assessment of radioactive fallout from Chernobyl, examining in particular the different forms of knowledge drawn on by the farmers (Wynne 1989). The Lake District received some of the highest levels of fallout in Western Europe, and as a result many farmers were not able to sell their stock (ibid.). Wynne looks at the different forms of knowledge drawn on by farmers. For example, farmers were aware of the different soil types at different sites, which had consequences for whether radiocesium would be immobilized in the soil and whether it would be incorporated in new growth. Scientists were initially unaware of, or indifferent to, this local knowledge and assumed that the farms were standard, thus ignoring what could potentially be significant variations between them. Scientists made corresponding statements as if their knowledge was certain, eliding the complexity of the farmers working conditions. Farmers were far less certain, and indeed were used to a degree of uncertainty due to the nature of the work and the often unpredictable conditions. In response to the arrogant approach of scientists, farmers became very dismissive and untrusting of their 'expertise'.

Economic and social pressures can have a major impact on the willingness of people to expose themselves to risk. These are often ignored by experts, or are unable to be included in their models for assessing, and dealing with, risk. Wynne provides the illustration of this with radiation workers who were supposed to use exposure-recording instruments that would indicate when they had reached the official dose limit. These instruments were removed by workers so that the dosage would be under-recorded in order to avoid the workers being shifted from work that attracted bonuses (Wynne 1987). Radiation workers at the Sellafield reprocessing plant exposed an unsuspected 'positive social construction of ignorance' (Wynne 1995). Here, workers made deliberate decisions to remain ignorant about certain issues, such as radiation risks, justifying their ignorance on a number of grounds. First, if they started to follow the dispute about risks, they felt it would be unproductive and ongoing. Second, it would mean confronting endemic uncertainties which would be both unsettling and dangerous. Third, to show an active interest in the topic would signal a mistrust of those experts who were meant to protect them. Thus Wynne's studies cast doubt on the credibility of expert risk analysis. Experts assume that ideal conditions are met, whereas in reality they will only be met in the appropriate economic, political, social and cultural circumstances. At the same time workers actively choose to be reliant on experts, as the costs of not doing so are too high.

Public health experts and scientists may play a role in identifying and publicizing risks, but there are many instances where it has been left to lay people to have the issue appropriately dealt with. An illustration of this is Robinson's discussion of the exposure of Californian workers to dibromochloropropane (DBCP) pesticide (Robinson 1991). In the 1950s, scientists had found that DBCP had reproductive toxicity in laboratory animals. The scientific evidence was published in 1961. As a result, several government agencies investigated DBCP but no further action was taken. Then, in the 1970s, a number of Californian workers involved in the manufacture of DBCP were found to be sterile. The union, once alerted to the possibility that this was caused by DBCP, took the action of collecting and evaluating semen samples of the workers. The chemical company denied the union's request for a hygiene evaluation. The union was able to get a national regulatory agency interested, but only after the media had already expressed interest in the issue. It was soon found that other workers from Colorado, Arkansas, Israel, Costa Rica and Mexico had also reported sterility, and not long after, DBCP-contaminated water supplies were identified and residues were found on fruit. The Environmental Protection Agency then banned the pesticide. Those who blew the whistle on the dangers of DBCP were not the managers of the companies producing it, not the corporate scientists, and not the governmental regulating agencies – but the workers themselves (Robinson 1991).

There is, it can be argued, something in the nature of science that means that it is not adept at identifying new potential risks. Scientific theory enables phenomena to become understandable by drawing attention to very specific aspects of the world around us. But in doing this, it also means that many aspects of the world are not attended to, and so escape being rendered intelligible. The knower, or scientist, is actively involved in the construction of knowledge which is therefore not simply a neutral reflection of the surrounding world. An example that supports this perspective is the measurement of ozone depletion. In 1985 NASA confirmed ozone losses over the Antarctic which had been announced by a group of British scientists. But ozone depletion had, in fact, been recorded for some time, without it being 'discovered'; the computers responsible for recording and analysing data on ozone were programmed to discount drastically low measurements as erroneous (Weiss 1993). This was because the accepted models of polar atmospherics did not allow for such drops in ozone; so even though the ability to measure ozone depletion was there, the conceptualization of atmospherics prevented it from being seen.

Furthermore, even where a particular issue has been identified by the scientific community it does not follow that action will immediately be taken. Beck's concept of organized irresponsibility helps explain why this is so. Organized irresponsibility is an outcome of the inability of science to provide standards of proof upon which policy decisions can be based. Once the causative agent of a problem has been identified, it is then possible to intervene legally. But, since the legally acceptable standard of proof linking a possible agent to a particular illness is so difficult to obtain, perpetrators of pollution and contamination are, in effect, protected. In other words, the burden of proof is so high that perpetrators of pollution can avoid responsibility for their actions, thus bureaucratic laws 'transform collective guilt into general acquittal' (Beck 1995: 2).

Beck also states that individuals are constrained by the system within which they operate, influencing how they accept risk and how they determine the level of acceptable risk for others. Individuals can carry out tasks without having to take personal responsibility for the consequences, since they are simply acting in accordance with the system in which they operate. It is as if one were acting while being personally absent; one acts physically, without acting morally or politically. The generalized other, the system, acts within and through individuals; this is conceived by Beck as the slave morality of civilization (Beck 1992). There are those who dismiss risk, even when they themselves are in danger: 'As the hazards increase in extent, and the situation is subjectively perceived as hopeless, there is a growing tendency not merely to accept the hazard, but to deny it by every means at one's disposal' (Beck 1995: 48). In a study of the victims of Seveso (a fire in a chemical factory that contaminated local inhabitants with dioxin) Beck notes that locals accepted the statements by officials that played down the dangers, and bitterly criticized those who stressed the toxicity of dioxin. For Beck, this is clinging to normality in the face of intolerable contradictions.

When a potential risk has been identified, discussions between experts and concerned lay people are often unproductive. Hannigan illustrates this with his concept of 'toxic talk' in public meetings between authorities and concerned social groups (Hannigan 1995). Lay people are often bombarded with technical information, yet the information they want is not available. Presentations by experts are abstract, impersonal and technical, creating an impression of professional neutrality. If the public becomes angry and confrontational, they are dismissed as being 'emotional'. Overall, therefore, meaningful dialogue is impossible.

Scientific ethics is also ill-equipped to deal with such issues. As Beck argues, 'In the model of the objectified sciences, ethics plays the part of a bicycle brake on an intercontinental aeroplane' (Beck 1995: 119). What is needed, Beck suggests, is the development of a public sensitivity to risks, which must be articulated by social movements or some other vehicle for criticism and protest against science and technology. A new method for dealing with risks, for relating to risks, must be forced upon the sciences, a method that is not intrascientific, but is rather based on social definitions and relationships (Beck 1992).

There are, however, contrasting cases where it has been scientists that have highlighted uncertainties and the public who have downplayed the risks. An example is the release of the Rabbit Haemorrhagic Disease Virus (RHDV) in New Zealand in the 1990s. Farmers, whose land was being devastated by an uncontrollable plague of rabbits, had requested that the virus be imported from Australia as a biological control. The scientists responsible for advising the government on the matter invoked the precautionary principle, and the burden of proof that the virus would not cause unintended environmental harm was placed on those who wished to introduce the disease. Farmers were unable to assure adequately that the virus would not damage native fauna or important livestock, and subsequently scientists advised that the virus should not be released.

Faced with economic pressures to keep marginalized farm land productive, farmers took the experimental use of RHDV into their own hands and illegally imported the virus into the country (Dew 2003). Livers of infected rabbits were placed in household blenders, creating a concoction known as a 'rabbit smoothie'. This was spread on rabbit bait, which was then dispersed on various farms. As such, the manufacture and dispersal of the biological control was undertaken in hazardous circumstances that had never been assessed for its risks.

The farmers were using the virus as a biocide, something that had not been trialled before. Outside of New Zealand, the virus had previously been used as a biocontrol, being released into the environment and left to spread naturally. By invoking the precautionary principle, scientists were, in this case, emphasizing the uncertainty of risks, whereas farmers were much less cautious.

While Beck's characterization of risk society illustrates that contemporary hazards are a risk to us all, it does tend to ignore that some groups are more at risk than others. Murphy argues that we should develop categories of environmental 'classes' to supplement the sociological notions of economic and social classes (Murphy 1994). For Murphy an analysis of environmental classes will reflect the benefits and costs accumulated by different groups in their participation in environmental degradation. Some classes of people are actively involved in perpetrating environmental degradation with little cost – the private sector and the state, for example – while others are victimized classes. The state may be involved through acts of commission (such as the construction of power stations, or participation in military conflicts such as the environmentally destructive Gulf War) or omission (for example, not regulating the private sector effectively and therefore allowing them to degrade the environment). Obviously, some states are more exploitative of the environment than others, an example being industrialized nations dumping carbon dioxide into the world's atmosphere.

The victimized classes, such as the workers illustrated above, can be differentiated. First-party victims are those whose jobs involve exposure to hazardous substances, such as the 'glow boys' who go into radioactive areas to do repair work and chemical plant workers who are not compensated for cancer. Those who live in environments which are polluted by factories are also first-party victims. Second-party victims are those who choose to be in the system and therefore voluntarily accept risk. Examples of this might be those who use fuel for automobiles that contain cancer-causing elements. Third-party victims are those who do not actively participate in the system but nonetheless suffer from it: cyclists inhaling benzenes, for instance. And, foetuses who suffer from the degradation of either of their parents' environment, can be classed as fourth-party victims (Murphy 1994).

Dealing with a world characterized by risk, where some groups are faced with hazardous working and living conditions, is complicated by the difficulty of creating an awareness of particular risks. Cultural resonances are important in the public assessment of what is risky or hazardous (Hansen 1991). Particular environmental and public health issues experience considerable ups and downs both in the media and in public perceptions. The mass media is particularly important, and in order to understand its role in the elaboration of public health and environmental issues, we must, according to Hansen (ibid.: 444), 'recognise the importance of cultural resonances in the privileging of some issues over others'.

The mass media serve as primary sources of information, however, as commentators have made clear for some time now, the media do not simply transmit messages to a passively receiving public. For an issue to gain media prominence it must resonate with widely held cultural concepts (Hansen 1991). Hannigan (1995) looks at the construction of environmental controversies. He does not assume that there are no objective conditions of pollution, but rather he suggests that images and linkages need to be 'constructed' in order for an issue to become more dramatic and intelligible. Acid rain, for instance, was identified back in the nineteenth century, but no action was taken until the 1960s when it was linked to the death of fish in the lakes of Scandinavia. Similarly, the ozone hole is not a hole as such, rather a thinning in concentration, but the image of a hole gives dramatic impact and mobilizes action. Consequently, hazards may be overlooked if they fail to resonate with cultural sentiments.

The Settling of Risk Controversies

There is some variability in the trajectory of risk controversies when the courts are involved. Courts deal with confrontations between popular epidemiology and those arguing for a high standard of proof in different ways. For example, with the U.S. Vietnam War veterans the issue of causation took a different turn in the courts. In the case of Agent Orange in the U.S. the chemical companies involved in its manufacture reached an out-of-court settlement with the Vietnam veterans of $180 million (Hall 1989). When controversies are settled out of court they do not provide a precedent for other cases and responsibility for any hazardous exposure is not admitted. Additionally, in the U.S. the courts tend not to work on the basis of a null hypothesis, but base decisions on the weight of evidence. Such recourse to the courts is not available in all jurisdictions.

When medical issues come before the courts, there is discretion as to how the court systems will determine whether someone is suffering from a condition, whether that condition was caused by some environmental or industrial pollutant in question, and whether someone can be found culpable for the problem (Phillips 2009; Phillips 2010). Phillips looks at the case of multiple chemical sensitivities (MCS), noting that in some jurisdictions, such as Germany and Austria, a diagnosis of MCS is accepted. In others, like Western Australia, the diagnosis is not generally accepted by either the medical profession or the legal profession. Even in the same jurisdictions, cases can be treated differently before the courts, with some courts being convinced on the balance of probabilities of a particular diagnosis, its cause and who is culpable, and others relying on more stringent medical definitions of causation – closer to a notion of absolute proof. Courts might accept testimonial evidence, that is, what people suffering from a condition have to say, but more often than not, testimonial evidence is discounted as a means for proving causation. There is, as Jasanoff would say, no accessible, 'perfect, objectively verifiable truth' that can be used to settle such disputes (cited in Hannigan 1995: 91). Indeed, the way in which public health controversies are settled has a lot to do with political and legal influence, as well as persistence.

Science, therefore, is not able to play the role of an objective arbiter in determining risks or attributing causality and responsibility. Indeed, just how controversies concerning risk get settled can really only be understood by relating them to wider political and social phenomena. There is a strong resonance here with the position of actor-network theory (ANT). Latour argues that facts do not settle a controversy: rather, facts are the product of a controversy that has been settled. In other words, what we come to see as a 'fact' occurs at the end of the dispute over the nature of the world, it does not determine the outcome of the dispute. As a controversy plays out, whether it is in scientific circles or in a more public arena, various actors align themselves with particular sides. As an alliance builds a statement starts to resemble a fact (Latour 1987). Science is particularly adept at building such alliances and constructing facts because the costs of challenging specialized and expensive laboratory findings exceed the capabilities of any potential dissidents. Often, individuals or groups will identify with a potential fact that aligns with their own projects. In effect, controversies are settled in a way that reflects particular cultural formations. Specific controversies are settled differently, and science and scientists play varying roles.

Because of the high standard of proof required by scientists they become useful allies for state and business interests in denying culpability for the untoward outcomes of chemical and other exposures. This is illustrated in the case of timbermill workers in New Zealand who alleged that their long-term health problems (and the high number of deaths amongst their colleagues) were a result of exposure to a timber treatment chemical – pentachlorophenol (PCP). PCP was first introduced in 1936 for use as a wood preservative. Commercial grades of PCP used in New Zealand contained toxic impurities created during manufacture, including dioxin (Bingham 1992).

When workers attempted to get compensation for their illnesses, most were denied this on the grounds that there was no absolute proof that their conditions were related to PCP. Epidemiologists gathered information that indicated that there might be a connection between illnesses suffered by timbermill workers and the use of PCP, but they could not unequivocally prove this. This inability to get absolute proof was used to support the case of the timber industry and state authorities to deny compensation to workers (Dew 1999b).

A report from a National Task Group, set up to report on PCP- contaminated sites, stated that even full-scale epidemiological studies would be unlikely to distinguish cases of chemical exposure from symptoms arising from other causes, such as lifestyle and consumption behaviour impacts, hereditary conditions, and exposure to chemicals outside of the workplace (National Task Group 1992). There were obstacles to achieving scientific validation for the workers complaints: for example, the cost of measuring dioxin levels in the blood and the fact that a litre of blood needed to be taken, which was often too much stress for sick workers. Many of the sickest workers, who perhaps provided the best example of a link between chemical exposure and illness, had died and could not become part of the investigation. To complicate the picture, workers had, throughout their employment, been exposed to a range of chemicals, any combination of which may have exacerbated symptoms. Determining the effects of long-term exposure to a range of chemicals was an impossible task for science.

This case demonstrates that a number of problems are faced by occupational and public health physicians in determining causation. This is further exacerbated by a lack of information on occupational and environmental toxins. A working party, set up by the Royal Australasian College of Physicians to look at assessment in cases of chemical exposure at work, commented on the dearth of information available on chemicals. They noted that the Californian Public Health Department has some risk data on less than 10 per cent of the approximately fifty thousand chemicals in common use in California, and comprehensive risk data on less than 0.1 per cent of those chemicals (Gorman and Dryson 1998).

The lack of information about the actual formulations used and the degree and nature of contamination further compound this. There is also a concern that the diagnosis of occupational illness itself can have adverse effects on patients: 'the negative health effects, in part, are due to the profound aggravation of morbidity that often accompanies compensation' (Gorman and Dryson 1998: 35). Underlying this position is an assumption of the malingering worker with psychosomatic disorders seeking compensation. Judgements about the malingering worker conceal social and class prejudices, and where the issue of worker compensation is raised these concerns about malingering are heightened (Dembe 1998). In the case of the timbermill workers, the indeterminacy of science meant that the resolution of the controversy was to limit the compensation claims of workers. Public health scientists are, then, unwittingly enrolled in support of this outcome.

Controversies can of course be resolved in different ways. The example of attempts to eradicate exotic pests provides insights into other features of controversy resolution, including an important temporal dimension. Drastic measures to curb insect infestations can occur because of economic or public health concerns or, alternatively, can be the cause of public health concerns and the development of popular epidemiology social movements. In large populated areas (Vancouver in 1992, Victoria in 1999, Seattle in 2000 and Auckland in 2003) spraying of chemical formulas has been undertaken in an attempt to eradicate moths that have been identified as a threat to vegetation and forestry. These attempts to stave off economic ills incidentally generated a great deal of concern for health among the public.

In Canada, a patented spray known as Foray 48B was used to eradicate the gipsy moth and the painted apple moth. It was known that the spray contained

Bacillus thuringiensis, but the other ingredients were not disclosed by the manufacturer (van Netten et al. 2000). After the spray had been released using a fixed-wing aircraft, reports of adverse reactions started being made, with telephone hotlines receiving thousands of calls. Groups opposed to the spraying, such as STOP (Society Targeting Overuse of Pesticides), became involved. Research on those who lived in the spray zone revealed many concerns, not only worries about the immediate impact of the spray, but also how it might impact upon future generations (Hales et al. 2004). Even government-sponsored reports raised concerns about the limited ability of epidemiological studies to detect potential effects and contested the assumptions of studies that were used to reassure the public (ibid.). For example, Foray 48B is released from aircraft as a bioaerosol, which is a very fine suspension of biological matter in the air. The epidemiological studies used to reassure the public of the safety of Foray 48B did not take into account the effects of the spray when it was in this fine, mist form (ibid.). Bioaerosols, for instance, have the potential to be ingested much more deeply into the respiratory system than heavier particles, and this could account for some of the respiratory conditions that had subsequently been noted.

When concerns about the health impacts of spraying a population are raised, governments can call for research in order to defer making decisions. In the case of aerial spraying over Auckland in 2003, residents in the spray zone embarked on the classic popular epidemiological approach and began collecting information about adverse effects of the spray. Common symptoms reported included headaches, asthma exacerbation, diarrhoea, vomiting, malaise, swollen glands and skin rashes. The government of the day commissioned the report that raised concerns about the effects of the spray as a bioaerosol (Hales et al. 2004). This report, however, was not officially released until the spray programme was near completion, and government rhetoric implied that the report had concluded that spraying was safe. A press release from the Ministry of Health stated that 'it is important to note that this theoretical risk did not lead the authors to recommend stopping or modifying the existing spray programme' (New Zealand Ministry of Health 2004). The public health researchers who compiled the report were not permitted to make such a recommendation; it was not in their research contract to do so.

So again we can see public health researchers inadvertently embroiled in a process that might not lead to a 'just' outcome – in this case they were deployed to ensure the completion of the spraying programme. Even though their report raised questions about the spray, it was released at such a time, and framed in such a way, that the programme could be completed.

Another example of epidemiology being used unwittingly is the case of a group of firefighters who, in 1984, fought a fire at an ICI warehouse in Auckland, New Zealand, that was packed with chemicals (Dew 2002). Immediately after the fire, firefighters experienced a variety of symptoms, many of which lingered on; and by 1990, as many as 214 firefighters had reported health problems. There were complaints about a lack of compensation and so a commission was set up to investigate. An epidemiological study was undertaken, comparing ICI firefighters with firefighters in another city. This showed a significantly higher self-reporting of health problems in the ICI group, poorer neuro-psychological test results, and a higher incidence of ongoing skin complaints and central nervous system symptoms (Elias et al. 1990). The Commission, however, saw major problems in such a study, arguing that the lack of exposure data, the long latent period, recall bias, the problem of finding normative controls and the possibility of other confounding causes, meant that there was sufficient doubt as to the cause of the symptoms. The Commission concluded that there was 'no known toxicological justification' for an explanation of chronic skin or central nervous system symptoms experienced by firefighters following the ICI fire (ibid.). The Commission report stated that although the firefighters' symptoms were real and not imaginary, and although the firefighters suffered symptoms from exposure to toxins at the time of the fire, the symptoms that the firefighters continued to experience were due to stress and anxiety. These, it suggested, should improve with the alleviation of that anxiety (ibid.).

We can contrast the Commission's rejection of toxic exposure as a cause of illness with the willingness of the Commission to embrace the findings from a psychiatrist's report, despite the latter's much lower level of rigour. The psychiatrist's report noted the problems of a diagnosis of neurotoxicity and the lack of international standards for such tests. It went on to criticize an academic ecologist and Greenpeace for generating a sense of anxiety, and it also looked at past studies which concluded that fear and anxiety may have contributed to symptoms where health problems developed after handling chemicals. A very small study involving eleven Australians diagnosed with post-traumatic stress disorder was used to support the notion that the stressful event itself is relatively unimportant, compared to the prior psychological problems of the individuals involved. Other reports were cited that link the health of firefighters to the levels of stress they commonly experience, and others which concluded that 'disability following a working accident was primarily motivated by financial gain' (Elias et al. 1990: 280). The psychiatrist also found of great interest an incident of a fire involving pesticides, herbicides and insecticides where no firefighters were hurt. This led the psychiatrist to conclude that the symptoms were a result of 'chronic and unfortunate stress' (ibid.: 291). The report of the psychiatrist was essentially a collection of loosely associated ideas linking anxiety to the symptoms, and by no means presented an epidemiologically demonstrable link between stress and the particular symptoms experienced by the firefighters. Yet, despite this uncertainty about the causal link, it was from this report that the Commission drew its conclusion and confirmed that anxiety and stress were the cause of the ICI firefighters' ills.

In their recommendations to deal with the 'anxiety' suffered by the firefighters, the Commission proposed an extension of the activities of the Occupational Health Service. It said that psychological counselling should be provided to all of those firefighters who seek it for the effects of stress, and that the Occupational Health Service should 'provide education in skin hygiene and treatment' to those firefighters who continued to suffer skin rashes (Elias et al. 1990: 109). It also proposed that all firefighters should undergo a number of medical tests at regular intervals.

This outcome had the potential to add further stress to firefighters. By being subject to a greater level of medical surveillance, it was more likely that firefighters could lose employment due to medical criteria. This outcome parallels Turner's Foucauldian analysis of the lobbying for safety legislation by workers in the mining industry. In Turner's example, the result of lobbying was a greater loss of worker autonomy. When safety legislation failed, it led to more legislation that increased the power of management (Turner 1989). Nelkin and Tancredi (1994) have noted that an increased testing of the workforce can exacerbate social disadvantage. They argue that the increased preoccupation with testing reflects an actuarial mind-set, which thrives on information about health, habits and behaviour. Nelkin and Tancredi go on to argue that there are incentives to test for the 'hypersusceptible' individual in the workplace, as there would be no need to change the workplace to make it safer – but attempt to identify and exclude the most susceptible workers (ibid.). Again, this resonates with the Commission report, where firefighters were constructed as overly anxious individuals and in need of better hygiene regimes.

What the ICI case illustrates is that the criteria for accepting a particular agent as causal are flexible. Anxiety, although not demonstrated with any certainty to be the cause, is quickly accepted as causal, whereas the epidemiology report, also lacking certainty but nonetheless demonstrating a possible link, was dismissed. The actual cause may have been stress and anxiety, and it could also have been from dioxin or a mix of this and other chemicals. But if the ICI chemical fire was proven as the cause and the state was, consequently, going to provide compensation, then the standard of proof had to be certain. This case demonstrates the elaborate mechanisms that give the semblance of rigorous analysis in order to produce outcomes that are favourable to all except the victims of injury.

What we see in such cases as the aerial spraying and the firefighters and timbermill workers exposed to chemical hazards is a particular, and at times unwitting, role that public health researchers and epidemiologists play. In these cases public health further victimizes the victims. State and business interests can use the high standard of proof required for identifying causality as a means of dismissing the claims of those exposed to hazardous substances – so 'business as usual' can continue.

The role of science in assessing causality is also complicated by variation in the burden of proof in different jurisdictions. In New Zealand, and the U.K., the standard of proof when assessing workers' compensation claims is very high; it is assumed that the illness in question is not caused by work factors unless, as we have seen, it is proven with certainty. This is by no means universal, however. In some jurisdictions, such as Ontario, Canada, it is the other way around; the hazard in question is assumed to cause disease unless it is proven otherwise (Watterson 1999).

These examples support Wynne's contention that uncertainty is actively created. Uncertainty is not simply the result of a lack of precision in our measurement of the objective world, but is actively created out of contending, conflicting cultural backgrounds and institutional projects (Wynne 1987). Abraham, in his study of drug regulation in the U.K. and the U.S., shows how regulatory agencies can award the benefit of the doubt to commercial interests, and that any uncertainty in the science can justify regulatory inaction (Kohler-Moran et al. 1995: 177). Coburn notes that the idea of an impartial, 'neutral science' can lend itself to business interests (Coburn 1999). The inability of neutral science to establish proof can converge with state and business interests to minimize the cost of accident insurance. This convergence is made particularly easy when disease is constructed by biomedical discourse as arising from one causative agent (Daykin 1999), and the difficulty in establishing a cause with certainty can easily lead to the disease being dismissed.

It is clear then, that in matters of risk and hazards in the domain of public health, science does not represent some sort of arbiter. As Daykin notes, 'decisions about such issues as occupational exposure levels and threshold limit values reflect value judgements about acceptable levels of risk and not just the rational application of scientific information' (Daykin 1999: 7).

Science can seldom provide the certainty required to determine causality, and this uncertainty can allow hazards to persist and culprits to avoid responsibility. The settling of controversies is well and truly a social affair; science is involved, but so are political and legal interests, and access to financial resources. For a hazard to become an issue, it must first resonate with cultural themes. Salient to the argument made here is that public health research is readily called upon to support vested interests.

Discussion

Public health researchers can mediate between communities and the state, but conversely may act as a buffer between them to the frustration of the communities and potentially the researchers. As we have seen, in many instances there is a great deal of uncertainty surrounding the findings of epidemiology. The examples of workers facing hazardous conditions and populations experiencing mass pest-eradication programmes illustrates the problems this causes with the way in which scientific findings can be used. Such findings can be made to excuse inaction because nothing in science is certain. One way to deal with this uncertainty is to consider findings in relation to other relevant issues and come up with a view of the most probable cause of an illness, the 'balance of probabilities' approach. However, the approach used all too often is that a much higher standard of proof has to be attained before claims about the adverse consequences of hazard exposure are accepted. This is a 'beyond all doubt' approach, which, as Beck has pointed out, tends to allow perpetrators of pollution to avoid responsibility for their actions.

The public are caught in a dilemma. As Giddens notes, we have to trust in experts. Where there is a lack of full information, then we are left in a position of trust. Giddens (1990) suggests that the opposite of trust is not mistrust, but dread or angst. The consequences of not trusting can be debilitating. We will see in chapter 6 that a consequence of not trusting expert systems is to have to follow complicated debates and become as fully informed and educated about issues as possible. This is no easy task for any particular issue, and any idea of being able to avoid trust is impossible given the complexities of modern society.

It should also be borne in mind that attempts to eliminate risk may exacerbate hazards faced. Clark uses a number of examples to illustrate this (Clark 1980). One is the use of insecticides. In the period 1947–1974, insecticide use in the U.S. increased tenfold (as a response to the perceived risk of insects on crops). Over the same period, crop losses due to insect pests increased by a factor of two. Clark argues that this was mainly due to the efforts to eliminate natural variability. Canada tried to eliminate a spruce budworm that creates an epidemic every thirty years or more. The budworm defoliates the trees, killing a good proportion of the older forests, and then itself dies out. Young trees replace those killed off. In an attempt to protect the mature trees for commercial purposes, insecticides were applied. The consequence was that, under these relatively unvarying conditions of insecticide control, budworms spread and persisted in high densities making the forest and forest industry more vulnerable. The destruction of the natural cycle allowed a lingering persistence. There are of course many other examples of attempts to eliminate risk that have created other hazards, but the point here is that we cannot avoid risk or creating hazards.

In issues of public health, science has always had a legitimizing function. If public health measures are simply the application of good science, then the implementation of these measures is ostensibly justifiable, and other forms of legitimation such as consensus or democratic-based decision making can be avoided. But science is also founded on the ideals of progress and critique: valid scientific method must produce falsifiable hypotheses, and disproved hypotheses must be discarded. Public health and its methodologies are not, however, just science, but also a means of intervention and a mechanism for resolving disputes. The complex set of tasks that public health undertakes defies any simplistic view that public health equates with social justice. Even in situations where public health researchers are unwilling accomplices, they can indeed exacerbate injustice. This ambiguous character of public health, as both a science and a means of intervention or advocacy, will be discussed in more detail in the next chapter.

CHAPTER 6
Public Health Campaigns

Introduction

In 1772, Edward Jenner took pus from the blisters of a milkmaid and injected the pus into the eight-year-old son of his gardener. He then deliberately injected the boy with smallpox (Halliday 2007: 282). The boy survived, and from such ethically sound research the process of vaccination was born. Today, vaccines are the most significant intervention used in attempts to eradicate communicable diseases worldwide.

Chapter 4 showed how public health projects can conflict with the practices of general practitioners, such that uniform public health initiatives impose upon the flexibility required by primary care physicians and general practitioners to successfully conduct consultations. This chapter focuses more specifically on this standardized and uniform nature of public health in relation to populations at large, illustrating this with the example of vaccination campaigns.

There are many examples of public health interventions promoting uniformity, such as the pasteurization of milk and cheese, fluoridation of water, and universal vaccination programmes. In these examples public health has pushed for the universal treatment of a food, the universal addition of a substance to an essential commodity, and the universal application of a preventive treatment to healthy people. The population, however, is not a homogenous collection of individuals with uniform desires. Obviously there is a great deal of diversity in terms of beliefs and rationales. For example, some may argue against pasteurization, or the process of 'boiling up milk', claiming that many nutrients are lost (Jeffreys 1998: 253). Similarly, fluoridation has provoked debate, with some claiming that it causes disease such as osteosarcoma, and that its protective properties are overstated (see Martin 1991, for an in-depth discussion of the fluoridation controversy). Vaccines have at times also been seen as a toxic attack on the body which lowers the responsiveness of the immune system (Chaitow 1987).

As this chapter will argue, it is important to note that despite the claims of some public health advocates, many of these rationales that conflict with public health measures are not necessarily irrational. In fact, some public health activities are open to accusations of a type of irrationalism. A claim is not being made here that rational is the same as 'correct' or 'true', or that irrational is 'false'. The truth or validity of a claim about nature is not being judged here. The term rational is primarily referring to the process that people use in coming to a decision and acting. Actions can be based on values and emotions, but they can also be based on considered thought about the consequences of action. Vaccination campaigns offer a useful illustration. Firstly, vaccination campaigns frequently violate the principles of informed consent, often held as a requisite for protecting individual rights. In contemporary health practice there has been a great deal of attention paid to informed consent in relation to treatment plans for patients, the collection and storage of tissues samples, and so on (Datta and Kessell 2010; Leith 2007; Stewart and DeMarco 2005). But the issue of informed consent may be regarded quite differently by those running public health campaigns, where the very act of 'informing' may run the risk of undermining the goals of the campaign. So rather than rationally informing the population, public health campaigns can focus on appeals to fear and other forms of irrationality. In this analysis, people are not necessarily 'informed' but are instead persuaded to conform to public health values.

Secondly, in many ways the implementation of these campaigns can be judged to have failed to adhere to the principles of good scientific endeavour. Public health advocates become so convinced of the perceived merits of the public health measures that there are selective presentations of fact, or a particular 'spin' placed on presented information. The same process of selective presentations can be used by those who are opposed to vaccinations as well.

Where science and a commitment to a particular view of the world come together there can be untoward consequences, including deception. This has been demonstrated by scientific research itself. Research has shown that some doctors are so convinced that they know what is best for their patients that they are tempted to cheat in clinical trials. In a study of 250 allegedly randomized trials in the U.S. and Britain, where codes identifying control and treatment groups were poorly concealed (pinned on the wall in the organizer's office for example), the data showed that the experimental treatment was on average 30 per cent more effective than when the codes were kept strictly confidential. That is enough to make a harmful treatment appear effective (Cohen 1995). How can this be explained? The argument made is that those involved in the research are so certain that they are right to give the particular treatment that they will manipulate the evidence to ensure that it aligns with their view. Hence, a powerful commitment to a particular paradigm can motivate fraud (Bridgstock 1982). Paradigmatic commitments and the motivations that follow can equally apply to those involved in public health.

It is important to note here that it is the work of scientists themselves that often detects such paradigmatic commitments, although sociologists, historians, journalists and others have also played an important role in this. In an early work along these lines, Gilbert and Mulkay identify a number of different repertoires used by scientists in their talk. An empiricist repertoire, which is the one we see in medical and science journals, provides an account of the scientist as detached, using the validated procedures of science and being drawn to whatever conclusions emerge from the facts. On the other hand, a contingent repertoire is used when scientists talk to others, such as sociologists, where scientists with different views are seen as social beings with desires, interests and affiliations that influence their beliefs and work (Gilbert and Mulkay 1984; Wooffitt 2005).

The inherent scepticism of science and its methodologies can be used to uncover such things as fraud and deception in scientific work that might arise out of a commitment to certain values or an attempt to obtain some gain. How this is responded to once uncovered, whether it is ignored, praised or vilified, is a social process that provides a lens on the particular values of the scientific community and of the public at large.

Public health acts as a moral force in society. It is partly underpinned by science, but the powerful commitment of public health advocates means that it often goes beyond science. There are many aspects of public health as a moral force that can be seen as a positive; public health advocates take on the alcohol industry, tobacco companies and the food industry – acting as a restraint against pathological forms of capitalism. On the other hand, public health can tend towards absolutism: it can impose its views on everyone on the basis of an absolute belief in the universality of its own values.

There are no clear institutional mechanisms that encourage conversations between those with varying perspectives on public health campaigns that might temper public health absolutism. As such, the diverse positions in debates are not always heard or responded to. If informed consent is taken as an important value, then this complicates the collective efforts of public health. If informed consent is seen as an important ethical issue in public health, then mechanisms for ensuring some kind of collective informed consent when dealing with collective interventions like mass childhood immunizations need to be developed. It is not being claimed here that those who challenge mainstream or orthodox public health views are correct – but the challenge must be made, orthodoxy needs to be tested, and ideally there should be some sort of platform for an open exchange of views.

Vaccination Resistance and Rationality

Today there is a great variety of vaccines, many of which are incorporated into vaccination programmes for children. In some jurisdictions these are mandatory, while in others they are supported by strong coercive campaigns to increase the uptake of vaccination (Dew 1999a). New vaccines are added to the schedule on a regular basis. In addition to the core vaccines for mumps, measles, rubella, diphtheria, poliomyelitis and tetanus, more recent additions to national vaccine schedules have included ones for varicella, haemophilus influenzae type B, meningococcal meningitis and the human papillomavirus.

From a public health perspective vaccinations are a good use of resources, based on the calculations made relating the costs of the intervention to the perceived benefits that are conferred. However, those supporting the introduction of new vaccines have to convince the public and politicians of their value, and arguments put forward by policy makers can be, and are, contested. The introduction of Gardasil as a vaccine to prevent cervical cancer provides an example. A U.S. organization called 'Judicial Watch' disseminated information about the number of adverse reactions to the vaccine reported to the Vaccine Adverse Event Report System. The vaccine is given to girls aged 9 and over and, as Judicial Watch pointed out, the Reporting System had collected over three thousand reported adverse events including eleven deaths in 2007 (Nelson and Moser 2008). There is, then, often considerable debate around the merits of vaccines, implementation programmes, and potential adverse reactions.

Social science analyses of vaccination issues have traditionally promoted more effective uptake of vaccinations. An early example is the writing of Stern, who, in the 1940s and 1950s, attempted to explain the irrational motives and vested interests of those who resisted vaccination procedures (Stern 1968). This analysis assumed the efficacy of vaccination procedures, echoing the position taken in most of the medical literature where the focus of concern is on ways of improving vaccine delivery systems and reducing costs of the system (Bazeley 1989; Foege 1997; Izuretia et al. 1997; Lee 1996; McGrath 1989; Muraskin 1995; New and Senior 1991). These studies implicitly accept the medical model's claim to scientific truth, and attempt to liberate the development of science and medicine from hindrances imposed by society (Rosenberg 1986). Public health proponents argue that 'vaccine-preventable' diseases are the major cause of death in young children, without even having to name the diseases themselves. Such accounts assume an unproblematic relationship between the receipt of a medical intervention – a vaccine – and the public's protection from disease.

Some social science research on the rationales of vaccine dissenters has, however, generated different interpretations. Representations of vaccinations and disease vary according to the social location of different groups, with health promotion groups and dissenting parents taking diametrically opposed views (Rogers and Pilgrim 1995). Non-acceptors may have sound reasons for their stand and have the same concerns about protecting the health of their children as acceptors (Streefland 2001).

Resistance to vaccination in economically poor nations can be particularly strong. Editors of medical journals, for instance, have accused vaccine manufacturers of exaggerating the number of deaths that result from the absence of the relevant vaccine. Authors based at the Center for Disease Control in Atlanta admitted a 50-fold inflation of hepatitis B mortality in India (Puliyel and Madhavi 2008). More broadly, unease has been expressed over the way in which the WHO and UNICEF have imposed programmes on nations, with such an imposition being eagerly accepted by governments despite the lack of 'scientific' evidence to support them (Banerji 1990).

Those who question the merits of vaccination campaigns face formidable opposition. The practice of vaccination to confer immunity or protection from infectious disease is held in such high regard within both the medical community and the public at large that it is presented as a cornerstone of preventive medicine (Streefland 2001). Heller argues that there is a cultural narrative of vaccination, defining a cultural narrative as: 'An economical story that elides and overwhelms contradictions, and simplifies our understanding of reality with scripted meanings and metaphors so that we can more easily make sense of the whole' (Heller 2008: 8).

Due to the cultural traction gained by the view of vaccinations as the eradicator of deadly and debilitating diseases, they have become something of an icon of modernity (Johnston 2006). This is particularly so of the smallpox vaccine. This was the first vaccine to be widely used, and its success continues to encourage similar campaigns: the eradication of smallpox is often held as the prime example of vaccination, and it has become the basis of a vision of universal disease eradication (Copp and Zanella 1992). Indeed, it is suggested here that the hope of emulating this achievement and wiping other deadly diseases from the face of the earth has acquired so much strength and momentum that it allows for very little dissension: if there is a price to pay for some in terms of adverse reactions to vaccinations then that is for the good of the whole community, and ultimately the whole world.

The Exemplar of Smallpox Vaccination

The history of smallpox public health interventions paints a much more complex picture. In 1840, a Vaccination Act was passed in England that enabled the free vaccination of infants with a vaccine made from cowpox. The relatively benign cowpox, due to its similarity with smallpox, prompts an immune response that provides protection against both diseases. The Vaccination Act outlawed the use of variolation – this involved infecting someone with a 'mild' form of the much more dangerous smallpox (Halliday 2007). Edward Jenner, who developed the cowpox vaccine, had inoculated himself with smallpox, the variolation method, but became very ill as a consequence (ibid.). In 1772, when Jenner observed that milkmaids appeared to be protected from smallpox, he attempted the experiment noted at the beginning of this chapter. The result of this experiment was a widespread uptake of the vaccination method, and in 1807 Bavaria became the first nation to make smallpox vaccination compulsory (ibid.).

When Jenner first developed his smallpox vaccine there was no sophisticated blood screening and there was little knowledge of what was happening within the body as pus from pustules was forced into the blood stream. One consequence of this procedure was that other diseases were being spread through the population. Vaccines increased the risk of spreading hepatitis, leprosy and syphilis. These adverse consequences were not recognized at that time as the accepted belief held then was that an individual could only have one disease at a time; if someone had smallpox, they could not have any other disease. It was not until 1968 that there was any serious attempt to account for the risks of smallpox vaccine (Copp and Zanella 1992).

By 1801 the British Admiralty had ordered every person in the fleet to be vaccinated. Not to be outdone, Napoleon vaccinated his army in 1805 and consequently Jenner was showered with awards for services to humanity. It is interesting to note here that it was armies and navies that first embraced Jenner's method. During the Napoleonic wars, Britain was facing mutiny from its navy which was demanding more money and more health services, and it may have been fortuitous that Jenner's method occurred at this time.

However, resistance to vaccination in Victorian England was strong, particularly from the working class, who interpreted vaccinations as a violation of their bodies and as a form of political tyranny (Durbach 2000). By looking at the historical detail of incidences of resistance to vaccination it is apparent that these are not simply irrational responses. In 1871, in Islington, London, a man named only as Jones was sent to prison for failing to present his child to a vaccination station (Barrow 2002). The compulsory vaccination laws of the time meant that Jones was required to bring his child to the station for the poor, to receive lymph vaccinations from another child. Here, a practice of arm-to-arm vaccinations was used, where lymph from the sore of a baby vaccinated a week earlier was used to vaccinate other babies. In the first instance, Jones diligently followed this provision. However, the compulsory vaccination laws also made it mandatory for selected children to return a week later to check if the vaccination had worked and to determine whether a child should be a vaccinifer – a child whose lymph would be used to vaccinate other children presenting that day.

Jones did not present his child for this second surveillance visit as he was told by his local medical officer not to; there was a child dying of smallpox in his house, making him and his children at risk of spreading the disease to others. The vaccinator took the case against Jones as his child was the only potential vaccinifer for that week, and so was the only one that could provide the lymph for the arm-to-arm vaccination process (Barrow 2002). The conditions of these poor stations could be deterrents to parental compliance. They were full of children who might be ill, and, as the above case illustrates, medical officers saw them as a means of spreading disease. It is not surprising then that in many jurisdictions there was little uptake of these regulations as the medical profession itself did not always support and enforce them.

Such examples usefully contrast the idea of the vaccination movement being rational and anti-vaccinators being irrational. Often in the literature on vaccinations, a picture will be portrayed of the heroic and rational vaccinators fighting off the irrational anti-vaccination lobby (Peckham and Hann 2010). This historical example described here foregrounds a different analysis; the view of anti-vaccination stances as a rational response to poorly administered and draconian laws.

Contemporary Rationalities

The apparent contrast between rationality and irrationality can be unsettled in contemporary society as well. Those who do not vaccinate their children can be characterized as falling into two main categories. In the first category are those from low socio-economic groups and ethnic minorities who do not receive vaccinations because the health services have failed to deliver to them. This group includes those from more inaccessible parts of a country that, due to the cost of transport, mean they are unable to get vaccinated. For this category, the received public health solution is to provide better, more accessible vaccination programmes. The second group, usually viewed as being very tiny, consists of 'conscientious objectors' – those who are unvaccinated as a result of a conscious choice (Hamilton et al. 2004), the worried healthy, the middle classes who have not experienced the terrible diseases of the past and have an irrational fear of vaccination. In the U.S., this group is reported to constitute as little as 0.3 per cent of the vaccination target population (Heller 2008).

In contrast to these analyses of rational versus irrational responses to vaccinations, New and Senior (1991) show how mothers draw on their past experiences of both vaccinations and diseases when it comes to making decisions in relation to their own children. In their study of vaccination uptake in the U.K., one mother was told that immunizations did not cause any side-effects, and so after her first child developed an allergic reaction to a vaccine she stopped vaccinating her children. Other mothers did vaccinate their children originally, but after their children developed the 'vaccine-preventable' disease, in spite of the 'protection' given, they ceased further vaccinations. This demonstrates that people do not passively receive the messages of health campaigns and health professionals; they assimilate information from a diversity of sources, including their own observations. Decisions based on this variety of sources of information can be seen as deliberative.

Those who do make the deliberate choice not to vaccinate often engage in a great deal of work to validate their position. Hobson-West provides a rare example of research on 'vaccine critical groups' in the U.K., such as the Vaccine Victims Support Group and Informed Parent. She notes that members of these groups undertake intensive reading of information from a wide variety of sources (Hobson-West 2007). To challenge expertise means that either other 'experts' have to be trusted, or you have to become an expert yourself: there is 'a strong moral imperative on the parent to become informed' (ibid.: 211).

Hobson-West provides further insight on how groups who have actively chosen to avoid vaccinations reach such decisions: some were worried about the objectivity of information provided by official sources; some believed that the benefits of vaccination had been overstated; some felt that vaccinations themselves create new health risks and that there are unknown outcomes from mass childhood vaccination (Hobson-West 2007). In her article, titled 'Trusting blindly can be the biggest risk of all', Hobson-West argues that instead of being ignorant and irresponsible, those who are 'vaccine critical' put a great deal of effort into being informed and taking responsibility. To do so means not simply trusting official sources of information, but critiquing that information, a stance that resonates with the concept of reflexive modernity discussed in chapter 5. It is much easier to be ignorant and to trust, because then you do not have to try to follow complex arguments and you do not have to take responsibility – you can relinquish such decisions to others. From this perspective, vaccination is the easiest option based on trust in expert systems.

Hobson-West argues that in order to understand resistance to public health measures such as vaccinations, we should consider them in relation to public perceptions of uncertainty. Mistrust of claims can develop due to a reframing of risk in terms of what we, as a society, do not know, or what we are uncertain about. We can link this back to a Durkheimian framework of public health as religion: dissenters critically interrogating the 'science' of public health, whilst public health campaigners minimize the unknown and uncertain elements of their practice in order to achieve the public health goals of mass vaccination.

Similarly, we can also consider resistance in terms of the construction of individual risks and uncertainty (an egoistic construction) versus constructions of collective risk. Collective constructions emphasize that some sacrifice must be made for the greater good. Research on vaccine resistance has found that parents who decline vaccines may construct risks at a personal rather than a population-based level. That is, the decision not to vaccinate may relate to concerns about the particular characteristics of their child such as a vulnerability to adverse reactions (Hobson-West 2007).

There are therefore contradictory moral forces at play. Using Hobson-West's work, we see that egoism, drawing on Durkheim's term, is not used in a negative sense. Rather, it refers to the notion that it is the particular situation of the individual (or his or her family) that is the prime consideration, and not the collective as a whole. Hobson-West eloquently summarizes this point when she states that vaccine resisters may 'construct trust itself as a source of risk' (Hobson-West 2007: 212). From the 'vaccine critical stance', it is not the case that parents should either trust official sources or trust the vaccine critical groups, but that parents should engage in a process of personal education in order to trust themselves. Here, it is trust in others that is a source of risk.

Immunization and Science

Individuals who actively refuse to take part in vaccinations, then, ought not to be simply dismissed as being irrational. Conversely, public health is not simply a rational, scientific endeavour. This can be demonstrated in regards to immunization campaigns, which, if we follow Karl Popper's prescription for science, are not falsifiable; whatever happens as the result of a campaign can be explained away without having to modify the beliefs that justify immunization. In other words, there is no outcome that would prove the theories underlying immunization as false, and so there are no grounds for contesting immunization campaigns.

A particular focus of Popper's was on the problem of demarcation in science, that is, what distinguishes a science from a pseudoscience. He was the Professor of Logic and Scientific Method at the University of London, and in his book *The Logic of Scientific Discovery* he claims that one cannot verify a hypothesis (such as, for example, that all swans are white) as there may be, at any time, an observation that proves it wrong. For Popper there was no such thing as certain knowledge, but we could support a hypothesis on the condition that it could potentially be proven wrong, as long as it had, up to that point, not been proven wrong by testing. Such hypotheses are said to be 'falsifiable'. Although they do not constitute absolute, certain knowledge, the more times they are not proven wrong by testing, the more certain they become (Popper 1972).

Importantly, as Popper suggests, an 'Open Society' is required to provide the necessary social conditions for falsifiable science to exist. Such a society supports the open exchange of information and promotes friendly-critical debate. Open, friendly-critical debate ensures that hypotheses can be circulated and tested by peers. For Popper, science was dynamic and critical, and involved a collective enterprise of critique (Popper 1972).

Popper was especially concerned with the influence of three perspectives – astrology, psychoanalysis and Marxism – which he felt were encouraging beliefs and behaviours that had no scientific basis (Popper 1963). Marxism, according to Popper, was not open to falsification because any argument against it can be labelled as an outcome of false consciousness; and, any of Marx's predictions that are not fulfilled are accounted for by the further extension of capitalism and its self-supporting ideologies. Similarly, psychoanalysis and astrology would provide self-legitimating explanations for any findings that contradicted their theoretical positions on the world.

In some respects, immunization campaigns have exhibited more of the characteristics of astrology than of Popper's ideal of science. To illustrate this we can look at two moments in measles vaccination campaigns in New Zealand: a 1984/85 epidemic and a predicted epidemic of 1997. The first moment involves the concept of herd immunity; a very powerful concept that promotes efforts to obtain universal, or near universal, population coverage of vaccines (Hobson-West 2007). If a high enough proportion of a population is vaccinated, then it is believed herd immunity will be achieved as sufficient individuals are immunized so that any potential reservoir for the disease being targeted is abolished; the disease can therefore be wiped out. Even those very few individuals who refuse to receive vaccination will be protected. It is argued that if a significant proportion of the population is not vaccinated, then there will be a sufficient number of unvaccinated individuals susceptible to the disease which can then become the source of an epidemic at any time. Thus, if herd immunity is not achieved, it is only those specific individuals who have been vaccinated who will be protected and the disease will not be eliminated.

In 1981 in nearly all districts in New Zealand measles vaccination rates were over 95 per cent – the level at which it was believed herd immunity would be obtained and the disease would effectively be eradicated (Day 2008). This view of herd immunity was demonstrably undermined by the measles epidemic of 1984/85. But the initial blame for the epidemic, as noted in the national medical journal, was low immunization rates (ibid.). That is, it was thought that the vaccination coverage was well below the 95 per cent level required to reach herd immunity. After the failure to generate herd immunity became apparent, it soon emerged in the public sphere that the vaccination failure rate was around 30 per cent. So, a prediction had been made that an epidemic of measles would not occur if herd immunity was achieved, and this was thought to occur with a 95 per cent vaccination coverage rate. Yet, when it became clear that herd immunity had not been achieved, other explanations were provided in order to account for the lapse; the theory of herd immunity and the supposed corresponding benefits were unquestioned and retained. Astrologers may account in a similar way if their predictions do not come true: inconsistencies are explained away as being the result of an unforeseen astral influence, or an individual's incorrect birth date.

In this instance the theories underpinning herd immunity and vaccination campaigns were saved by laying the blame for the epidemic on something being wrong with the actual vaccine. There were many aspects of vaccinations that could have been questioned: perhaps they do not confer immunity for as long as was thought and booster shots would be required, or it could be that there is something wrong with the handling and storage of the vaccines that made them impotent and so new systems for handling would have to be introduced. But, rather than question the accepted theory of vaccines in the spirit of scientific scepticism, such failures typically lead to calls for adding more vaccines to the vaccine schedules and further pressure to persuade the population to vaccinate (Dew 1999a).

We can contrast this case of a surprise epidemic with the next case, where an epidemic failed to appear as predicted. Mathematical modelling had predicted another measles epidemic, and so in 1997 the New Zealand Ministry of Health launched a measles vaccination campaign which included television and magazine advertising. The following is taken from public health advertising in *Women's Weekly*:

> We estimate that 45,000 New Zealand children will be hit by the Measles epidemic this year. Of these, four thousand will have ear infections, pneumonia or diarrhoea. Approximately nine hundred will be hospitalized. Thirty will suffer brain inflammation. Up to nine will be left with permanent brain damage. At least four will die. You have a choice. Talk to your doctor about free immunization and remove the risk of Measles forever. Or pray your child doesn't join the dots. Measles. It's not a pretty picture. (Cited in Dew 1999a)

Setting aside the disempowering message here – that if you do not immunize, all you have left is prayer – the predicted epidemic as described above did not occur.[1] Again, this did not lead to the questioning of vaccination theories and concepts like herd immunity. What these two examples suggest is that the theories which inform vaccination campaigns are not falsifiable. Many of the decisions being made in such campaigns are 'extra-scientific'; yet, they are being presented to the public as being purely objective.

Thus it can be argued that the idea of scientific scepticism, central to the scientific enterprise, is not followed in the arena of public health vaccination campaigns. As Paul Feyerabend argues, scepticism in science is not directed at currently-held views but:

> is directed against the views of the opposition and against minor ramifications on one's own basic ideas, never against the basic ideas themselves. Attack on the basic ideas evokes taboo reactions ... Basic beliefs are protected by this reaction as well as by secondary elaborations ... and whatever fails to fit into the established category system or is said to be incompatible with this system is either viewed as something quite horrifying or, more frequently, it is simply declared to be non-existent. (Feyerabend 1987: 305)

Vaccination dissenters evoking the taboo reaction can be described in the most acerbic terms. The New Zealand Department of Health's description of the Immunization Awareness Society (IAS), whose goal was to inform parents on all aspects of immunization, was 'a bunch of freaks, totally neurotic' (cited in Day 2008: 282). Andrew Wakefield, a researcher who had a paper accepted and published in *The Lancet* in 1998 claiming a link between the measles, mumps and rubella vaccine (MMR) and autism, not only was vilified as being dishonest and irresponsible, but had his paper formally retracted from the journal twelve years later and was banned from practising as a doctor in the U.K.[2] On receipt of the news of his ban, Wakefield stated that: 'It seemed to me that they had come to this decision a long time ago, long before the evidence was fairly heard. This is the way the system deals with dissent. You isolate, discredit and provide an example to other doctors and scientists not to get involved in this kind of thing. That is examining questions of vaccine safety' (Boseley 2010). Challenging the sacred elicits personal attacks and can have severe consequences.

There is no claim being made here that Wakefield was right and the medical establishment was wrong, or vice versa. What is of interest here is the reaction to the claims from the medical establishment. There are examples where scientists have clearly been identified as conducting fraudulent or unethical research and have not received the kind of response that Wakefield has. A well-known historical case discussed by Sapp is that of Ernst Haeckel, a late-nineteenth-century biologist and popularizer of Darwin's theory of evolution (Sapp 1990). Haeckel produced inaccurate drawings of embryonic development to confirm Darwin's theories. His frauds were exposed by creationists, but far from being disowned by the scientific community he was its champion – his frauds did not detract from his reputation. Why was this the case? According to Sapp, this was because Haeckel was on the side of the angels. Sapp suggests that every leading scientist could be found guilty of fraud in science if the standard is some objective methodological truth (ibid.). To illustrate, in the very same edition of the *British Medical Journal* that published an article outlining Wakefield's sins against the scientific community written by a journalist, an article appeared demonstrating the extent of bias in reporting outcomes from clinical trials. Of the fifty-nine clinical trial investigators interviewed, sixteen had failed to report outcomes that had been analysed and seventeen collected data that was not analysed. In many cases the failure to report outcomes was based on a view that the findings were uninteresting or were negative, or that the reader would miss the important message if all the data was reported. The following quote from a trial investigator whose response was regarded as a 'deliberate misrepresentation' is instructive:

> When we looked at the data, it actually showed an increase in harm amongst those who got the active treatment, and we ditched it because we weren't expecting it ... there doesn't appear to be a kind of framework or a mechanism for understanding this association and therefore you know people didn't have faith that this was a valid finding ... so we buried it. (Smyth et al. 2011)

In contrast to Wakefield, there is no moral outrage expressed about cases like this. We can surmise here that because the investigators were being orthodox, and not contesting accepted frameworks, there was no need for the vitriolic response that is received by those who do contest orthodoxy. That is, if you are a fraud, but orthodox, you might not receive the same kind of treatment as if you are unorthodox. Norms can and commonly are breached in science, but only on some occasions do these breaches lead to such moral outrage. An important component of the vaccine narrative, according to Heller, is that, 'When the narrative is challenged, it sometimes gains strength. Throughout the history of vaccination, the response to opponents of vaccination has reasserted the narrative in terms designed not so much to refute specific claims about vaccines, as to undermine their applicability' (Heller 2008: 14).

Informed Consent and Public Health

As mentioned earlier in this chapter, many countries temporarily adopted a compulsory approach to smallpox vaccination. Under such protocols informed consent is obviously meaningless. This started to change in the early twentieth century, when there was a movement from compulsion to persuasion (Day 2008). But, despite this general shift, in contemporary times there is considerable variability between different nation-states in terms of just how much force or persuasion is deployed when attempting to vaccinate a population. While in some states there is no overt compulsion, in others, individuals can only decline vaccination on religious grounds.

For example, in South Carolina in the U.S., a bill was considered in the 1960s to make administration of the poliomyelitis vaccine compulsory. Supporters of this bill stated that 'when the public refuses what is best for it ... the more resistant should undergo some legal coercion for the good of all' (Dubos 1965: 430). Similarly, the Australian Medical Association called for legislation that would allow exemption from vaccines only on the basis of a genuine medical contraindication (Rose 1991). This means that people would not be able to claim exemption on religious or philosophical grounds. Although these measures appear draconian, they can be justified by the different legislative bodies on the basis of international conventions. For example, the United Nations Convention on the Rights of Children obliges signatories to ensure the highest possible standards of health care for children (ibid.). The medical profession and health departments can argue that such conventions override individual rights.

Even in nations that have not reverted to overt compulsion, a 'compulsion by stealth' can occur. For example, in the 1920s the Department of Health in New Zealand regarded it as too difficult to gain informed consent from individual Māori for typhoid vaccination campaigns, and so instead sought to attain tribal consent. In order for this to be carried out, health department employees who had received tribal consent had to be indemnified by the government against charges of assault for vaccinating children without informing or gaining consent from parents (Day 2008). It was not until 1962 that the notion of tribal consent was dropped (ibid.). Unsurprisingly, typhoid campaigns were often labelled as racist. It was not unusual for Māori children in a school to be vaccinated against typhoid while their non-Māori schoolmates were not. Understandably this was seen as a racial slur against Māori (ibid.). The rationale for vaccinating Māori children was that they lived in poorer, less sanitary conditions than non-Māori, and were therefore more susceptible to typhoid. Vaccination was a cheaper or more politically palatable solution than improving sanitary conditions.

Public acceptance of vaccine programmes has not been helped by reports that children, particularly those who are most marginalized in society, have been used as guinea pigs for experimental vaccines. 'Minority' infants in Los Angeles and children in Haiti were used to test a vaccine which was eventually withdrawn because of an increase in the mortality rate of those babies who received the vaccine (Cockburn 1996). In a similar example of the targeting of marginalized groups, in Australia between the 1940s and 1960s vaccines were trialled on orphans (Reuters 1997).

The issue of informed consent also raises questions in relation to other aspects of vaccination implementation. In the 1960s, a polio vaccine known to be contaminated with the SV40 monkey virus was knowingly administered to millions of people in a number of countries (Martin 1996). The public had no knowledge that they were receiving a vaccine contaminated with a virus (Day 2008). Polio vaccines were cultured in the live kidneys of monkeys, making possible the contamination of such vaccines with unknown viruses that remain invisible as they may have no deleterious effect on their natural monkey hosts. The risks of such a procedure and the SV40 example have led one researcher, Louis Pascal, to suggest that contaminated polio vaccines, which were administered in mass immunization programmes in west and central Africa, are the origin of the AIDS pandemic (Martin 1996).

Biopower and Statecraft

The development of mass immunization programmes can be located within the dynamics of what Michel Foucault terms biopower, discussed in chapter 3. Foucault argues that one important dimension of the power over life which has been evolving since the seventeenth century is that of a biopolitics of the population. This focuses on biological processes: birth, mortality, health, longevity, and all the conditions that can cause them to vary. As Foucault suggests, these biological processes become regulated and in this way the state is strengthened (Foucault 1988).

When power is exercised on bodies it renders them as both the object and effect of knowledge (Nettleton 1985). People's lives become managed and knowledge is derived from them through a system of surveillance and normalization of bodies. 'Vaccine-preventable' diseases are threatening and therefore intervention and regulation is imposed to normalize all bodies. All bodies are to be made immune to the disease. A further transition meant that the viruses are no longer seen as the primary source of danger, but instead the individual who may transmit the disease, and therefore the individual had to be controlled.

The biopolitics of Foucault's Disciplinary Society incorporates and integrates technologies that reinforce each other. This can be illustrated by the example of the vaccination certification required in many countries for school entry purposes. Those who are recorded as being unvaccinated can be discriminated against and refused admittance to schools during epidemic outbreaks. These interventions can be seen in terms of the Christian metaphor of pastoral care, aimed at sustaining and improving the lives of everyone (Smart 1985), and so 'bio-power is spread under the banner of making people healthy and protecting them' (Dreyfus and Rabinow 1982: 195).

Increasing attention to vaccination uptake has grown in the Western world with the rise of the neo-liberal state. Osborne's view that in terms of statecraft the state cannot guarantee the health of the population was noted in chapter 4. A neo-liberal response to this is to determine the success of the state in the health area on the basis of quantifiable variables which become a 'surrogate' for health (Osborne 1997). In this framing, vaccination levels become important indicators of state success, that is, if vaccination levels are high the state has achieved its target. Medical policing of the population spreads out of the confines of public health itself. Structural incentives within health authorities, such as bonus payments to general practitioners for meeting vaccination targets, foster the downplaying of risks from vaccines to present a picture of safety (Ozonoff and Boden 1987). To claim uncertainty jeopardizes the goal of supporting policies of strong bureaucratic intervention (Britan 1981). By making certain aspects of social life, such as vaccines, sacred, these institutional structures place them beyond criticism (Herzfeld 1992). There is a transition towards a *polizeiwissenschaft* of health, where health is no longer a right of citizenship, but a duty of citizenship (Osborne 1997).

Alternative Views of Health

As we have seen from the above examples, those advocating vaccination campaigns often do so with a conception of health that is based on measurable aspects of populations. For public health, the intervention goal is quite simply measurable population-level declines in morbidity and mortality. And, when combined with health economics, the goal is how to do this in the most resource-efficient manner. As such there is no clear notion of what 'health' is within public health (in its epidemiologic manifestations). This population-based definition of health can, and indeed has been, challenged by those who take a different perspective on what actually constitutes 'health'. People conceptualize health in different ways and consequently can come into conflict with the more orthodox public health position.

There have always been diverse views on how best to promote and sustain health. Jean-Jacques Rousseau is credited with placing the *vis medica naturae* at the heart of the Romantic movement (Smith 2007). A call to go back to nature to live in an instinctual way, free from the fetters and constraints of society, was made under this rubric. For Rousseau, stringent habits and modern hygiene practices were just another constraint on living the good life. Rousseau advocated that children should be breast-fed, never swaddled, learn through play and fun, allowed to question freely, and live mainly outdoors: 'The only habit the child should be allowed to contract is that of having no habits' (cited in Smith 2007).

Ideas about what is natural for health could entail rigorous and sometimes unpleasant practices. In Roman times, hardening the body was a common practice among northern European tribes; children and babies were dipped into cold streams (Smith 2007). It was also a prominent notion in eighteenth-century Britain where hardiness was an essential part of hygiene (ibid.). A bracing cold bath was the favoured mechanism to bring about hardiness. These views of health, which conceptualize health and the 'good life' in terms that differ significantly from the position of current public health, resonate with some contemporary alternative views.

An example is those who valorize a more 'natural' state of life. Amongst some members of the population, and particularly those with an interest in complementary and alternative medicine, 'there is a widespread acceptance of things natural' (Coulter 2004). For some of these people, the closer one is to a natural state, the better off one is. This is in contrast to the public health perspective, where things natural are often considered threatening; being closer to a natural state may increase the risk of infections, or provide insufficient amounts of some vital or important element (such as fluoride or iodine).

Recently a perspective has developed in public health that mimics this appreciation of a more natural state. The hygiene hypothesis suggests that infections during infancy prevent the emergence of allergies and asthma later in life. In accordance with this argument, since children in the Western world are often kept away from the sorts of 'natural' conditions that cause such infections, asthma and allergies have become rife. The use of antibiotics, painkillers and other 'non-natural' agents, may also increase the risk of these conditions (Cohet et al. 2004). As such, the efforts to shield people from 'nature' are seen as having some negative consequences. Of course, what actually constitutes 'nature' varies in different debates, and the boundary between nature and culture can become somewhat indistinct. As White has pointed out, what might be seen as 'natural' in one time or place may, in another context, be seen as medical abnormality (White 1999).

The subject of harm to one's environment and to one's body that is posed by modern technologies raises the question of why people are prepared to take risks in some areas of their life but avoid risks in others. And what is it that makes one person take a particular risk while another person will avoid it? In the cultural theory of risk-taking, as developed by Mary Douglas, preferences among different types of risk-taking or risk-avoiding correspond to cultural biases, that is 'to worldviews or ideologies entailing deeply held values and beliefs defending different patterns of social relations' (Wildavsky and Drake 1990: 41). Therefore one's ideology or worldview will determine one's perception of risk.

Egalitarians claim that nature is fragile in order to justify sharing the earth's limited resources. Individualists claim that nature is abundant so that if people are released from artificial constraints, like environmental regulations, there will be affluence for all. Hierarchists approve of technological processes and products, provided experts have certified their safety, so good will follow from taking the advice of experts, and bad will follow if you do not. Thus the perception of danger depends upon the object of attention. Egalitarians may be most concerned about the risks of technology, but hierarchists are most concerned about social deviance, and individualists with the threat of war as it disrupts markets and imposes controls on people. So people perceive a different set of risks according to their ideology (Wildavsky and Drake 1990).

In an attempt to illustrate the variety of perspectives on health and what constitutes the 'good life', five positions can be noted: utilitarian, risk averse, realistic hedonist, purist and holist (Dew and Carroll 2007). It is not claimed here that these positions are exhaustive of all views on health, or that they are mutually exclusive. For any particular individual they could well overlap and people may change their perspective depending on circumstances. It is perhaps best to see these positions not as either/or, but as a continuum: people may adhere partly to one position, and partly to another. Each perspective will briefly be described here.

Utilitarianism is the 'orthodox' public health position whereby the focus is on increasing longevity and decreasing morbidity. Public health is based on this utilitarian value of the greatest well-being for the greatest number of people. From a population health perspective this means that on occasion some individuals may be required to suffer for the greater good, which is the well-being of the population: the overall quantum of health benefits will outweigh the quantum of suffering. This might characterize someone who chooses to immunize or not immunize, based on the contribution this will make to the community or population health.

The risk averse position has similar concerns to the utilitarian position, but in this case the focus is on the individual avoiding risks and suffering and not on overall population health gains. This might characterize someone who chooses to immunize or not immunize on the grounds of personal risks, such as a belief that they are particularly sensitive to adverse reactions.

A realistic hedonist perspective focuses on 'living life to the full', accepting that there is always a down side. Health is not conceptualized as the avoidance of disease; longevity, in itself, is not a goal. The issue of immunization is unlikely to have any clear relationship to this position.

A purist view may be concerned about longevity, but in this case the focus is on what is wholesome and pure. Contamination of the body is avoided, which includes the ingestion of toxic drugs. Immunization may be avoided due to a view that it introduces a toxic element to the body. Within this perspective, the body would be supported in a 'natural' way to fight off diseases. Vaccines may place 'stress on the immune system, rather than strengthening it' (Vernon 2003).

Holism is where one's individual health is only seen in relation to a broader dimension of environmental health. One's actions should enhance the environment and not cause damage. Both environmental and indigenous health beliefs align with this view. The focus on the environment may be related to protecting individuals, but is seen within the context of ecosystems. The issue of immunization may be quite complex in this position. It is possible that using vaccines may be seen as disrupting evolutionary principles or damaging the balance of life on earth.

Individuals or groups may incorporate different elements of these ideal types. It is possible that an individual can be utilitarian and risk averse or utilitarian and purist. But, at times, these positions can be in opposition, and in particular the population health perspective of the utilitarian model could clash with the realistic hedonist, holistic and purist perspectives.

These diverse perspectives on health have much wider ramifications than simply influencing attitudes to vaccinations. Attitudes to housing further demonstrate the impact of different understandings of public health. In one particularly illustrative study, interviews were conducted with people sleeping rough or living in a variety of types of informal housing, including garages, caravans and tents, old buses, house trucks and sheds (Carroll 2010). Those participants who were living in such conditions within a rural setting had made what they believed to be a positive choice to return to the land. They had rejected the comforts of urban life, and, from a public health perspective, were living in accommodation that is sub-standard: there may be no running water in their dwelling, no mains electricity, no insulation, no sewerage system. Instead, they used long-drop toilets, collected their water from a nearby stream or spring (and/or used rainwater off the roof), made do with candles and battery-powered lighting, and heated water and cooked on wood-fired stoves or with bottled gas. Many participants used a rhetoric of hardiness to describe their lifestyle: city living makes people soft and subsequently they have no real experience of living – living back on the land hardens you, makes you more resilient, and enhances your experience of life. Here, what many others may see as suffering and stress, is rearticulated as part of the process of 'toughening up' and gaining access to the experience of 'living life to the full' (ibid.).

These individuals rejected public health measures related to fluoridated and chlorinated water supplies, reticulated sewerage systems and septic tanks and mains electricity, although there was recognition that such measures could be necessary in an urban environment because of population density. For them, in their informal housing situations, such measures were often seen as unnecessary, wasteful of resources, polluting and expensive. Light and noise 'pollution' were highlighted as additional drawbacks to mainstream living. The preference for spring, stream or rain water rather than treated town-supply water was universal. In addition, those living in informal housing found the financial pressures of mortgages and rents unhealthy (Carroll 2010).

A utilitarian view of the relation between public health and housing is obviously at odds with these sentiments. From a mainstream public health perspective, the personal and public health risks of informal housing are readily identified. These risks include the unsafe use of gas bottles, candles and open fires; injury from living in structurally unsound dwellings; health risks from living in uninsulated, cold and damp dwellings; personal and environmental risks resulting from a lack of reticulated water and the use of alternative toilet facilities; and environmental problems caused by grey water discharge (discharge from baths and showers, from washing dishes, floors, clothes and so on).

The public health position supports a standardization of housing through codes and indexes. This overrides the range of views on what constitutes healthy living and the good life, many of which are affronted by the implementation of uniform public health measures.

Discussion

In sum, an orthodox public health perspective is utilitarian, with little exploration of the concept of health, a narrow focus in terms of measurement, and with the universal application of interventions and normalization of populations as basic goals. For those who dissent from the standardizing processes of public health a great deal of fortitude and commitment is required. To be informed is to be highly educated and resourced – and very few are in a position to be informed. It is very difficult for every individual to become informed and vaccine-critical – so some new institutional forms may better provide the chances of informed consent.

There is a history of 'lay' involvement in public health. In the early stages of public health, 'ordinary' people could participate in charitable and voluntary organizations aimed at improving the lot of the poor (Taylor 2007). For example, the use of health visitors to help the poor started off as a volunteer programme. 'Lay involvement' has been equated with 'active consumers' in the contemporary governance of health services, and it may also be used as a catchphrase to legitimate management decisions. But despite this, recently there have been attempts to procure lay input in the hope that the public will feel a sense of ownership over the resulting health service decisions (ibid.). Generally this has been in the context of programmes targeted at local communities, such as neighbourhood regeneration programmes. As yet there have been no noted examples of lay involvement in national decision-making processes related to services such as the implementation of vaccines. No doubt this is because health professionals see lay ideas of health and well-being as largely irrational (ibid.) and therefore having no place in a field of endeavour that is based on the science of epidemiology. But, as has been argued here, public health campaigns are not based solely on science. They are also about politics, paradigmatic thinking, values, and advocacy. The absence of lay involvement, then, should be queried.

At present, public health decision making in relation to population-based campaigns has little in the way of community input. There are no formal structures in which dissenting views can be aired, considered and responded to. However, an ethical framework prioritizing patient autonomy is a poor fit for public health practice (Gray et al. 2006). Public health workers themselves point out that there is no well-developed set of ethical principles or a framework that informs decision making of doctors working in public health (ibid.). In the absence of agreed-upon ethical frameworks, forums to bring opposing positions closer could be sought, in particular the opposition between personal autonomy and collective interventions. To insert diverse voices into public health campaigns complicates life for public health advocates – just as ethics committees complicate life for health researchers. But such short-term complications may ensure greater public trust in the long term.

The argument made in this chapter suggests that there are certain tendencies in public health that may need to be guarded against. Just as Durkheim suggested the need to counter the absolutist tendencies of the state, it is argued here that we should be similarly concerned about absolutist tendencies in public health and consider ways of countering them. If we are to move beyond trenchant opposition and we desire to build solidarity and trust, if our goal is the promotion of friendly-critical debate and an avoidance of hostile-paradigmatic positioning, then some forum to allow for this should be contemplated.

Notes

1. Other cases of failed predictions have occurred that have not led to changes in advice or policy. Heller cites the example of a severe 'flu vaccine shortage in the U.S. in the 2004/5 'flu season. Even the highest priority groups had a vaccine rate as low as 35 per cent. Not only did the expected crisis of hospitalizations and deaths from influenza fail to materialize, but the death rate was as good as or better than the previous two 'flu seasons (Heller 2008).
2. The article that *The Lancet* retracted was: A.J. Wakefield, S.H. Murch, A. Anthony, J. Linnel, D.M. Casson, M. Malik, M. Berelowitz, A.P. Dhillon, M.A. Thompson, P. Harvey, A. Vantine, S.E. Davies, J.A. Walker-Smith. 1998. 'Ileal-lymphoid-nodular Hyperplasia, Non-specific Colitis, and Pervasive Developmental Disorder in Children', *The Lancet* 351(3103), 637–41.

CHAPTER 7
The Cult of Health and its Rituals

Émile Durkheim predicted that a 'cult of humanity' will eventually take on the role played by traditional religions in premodern societies. This chapter pulls the threads of the argument in this book together by positioning public health as that contemporary religion – the cult of humanity (see Dew 2007 for an earlier expression of this argument). Viewing public health in this light explains the tensions of contemporary public health that have been explored in previous chapters, such as between advocacy and science, and equity and efficiency. Insight is provided into the uneasy relationship between clinical practice and health promotion. In addition, this view of public health positions it as a mediator between other powerful forces in contemporary society that foster, in varying ways, the excesses of capitalism (seen in endless consumption and lack of regulation). On the other hand, public health itself can be seen as a moral force supporting tendencies towards state absolutism, so in itself needs to be tempered. It is argued that within public health there are the 'seeds' of such a tempering that relate to the inherent scepticism of science, and public health holds in uneasy tension aspects of science and a cult or contemporary religion.

As noted in the opening chapter, Durkheim considered four contradictory moral forces in society: altruism, egoism, fatalism and anomie, with modern society characterized as one with an excess of egoism and anomie (Taylor and Ashworth 1987). Religion is one means of constraining these excesses. For Durkheim religion is a permanent feature of society (Mellor 2004) and an important form of collective representation that provides a function of cohesion and integration in society.

Durkheim predicted that in a modern society, with increasing social differentiation in a more complex division of labour, a cult of humanity would develop. This cult would take over the integrative function that traditional religions provided in the more undifferentiated earlier societies. Durkheim used the concept of organic solidarity to describe this increasingly diverse contemporary society, which he contrasted with the more undifferentiated form of mechanical solidarity that applied to societies where people were more homogenous and the chains and networks of interactions between people were less complicated. Durkheim contrasted the kind of work and interactions that would occur in a society comprised of small villages, where mechanical solidarity prevailed, with the work and interactions that occur in larger urban and industrialized settings, where organic solidarity prevails. In these very different societies, different kinds of religion would be evident.

With the irrepressible advance of individualism in modernity, worship would centre on the one thing that humans hold in common, their humanity (Westley 1978). Unity is a result of communal participation in religious activity and the communal acceptance of religious belief. Although religion would be performed in the individual's 'own heart' it would still have a number of social characteristics. This new religion would express the unity of society and hold periodic meetings where the values of society would be affirmed. The heresy of the cult of humanity is egoism, where individuals place themselves at the centre of worship.

Westley (1978) makes a number of predictions about the cult of humanity, which include: the cult of humanity will centre on the worship of common humanity, there will be religious diversification, sacred power will be seen to reside within the individual, religion and science will combine, and rituals will focus on the issue of purity. For one commentator the first dogma of the cult of humanity is the autonomy of reason, and its first rite is freedom of thought (Pickering 1984: 491). Humanist values require an authority that can be submitted to, and therefore Durkheim saw the necessity for the existence of a humanist religion. Human rights would be held sacred, and by the defence of these rights the fabric of society would be defended. The individual will be restricted and controlled by the imperative to respect the right of all other human beings (Westley 1978). The ambiguity between freedom of thought and the restrictions and controls on people links to the inherent ambiguity in human nature – described in the notion of *homo duplex*.

Durkheim deployed the concept of *homo duplex* to illustrate the state of tension for humanity between anomic desiring represented by the individual will, and the cohesion and constraint imposed by collective representations seen in societal institutions. This duality is inescapable. We are driven by our individual will but constrained by the social (Ramp 2003). Our will is irrational and based on biological needs and is in conflict with society (Mestrovic 1988). The will needs to be restrained for social order to exist. Public health in its variety of flavours can act as a restraint on both individual consumerist desires and the social and political environment that unleashes those desires.

To some it may seem far-fetched to see public health as a religion. Where is the spirituality? Where are the churches? But for Émile Durkheim, religion was not about spirituality and temples; it was a social practice that generates particular moral forces that help to sustain social order. Religion was 'not so much labels on a church building but the imagery seen in such things as myths and theology that people use to make sense of their lives' (Hammond 1974: 119). The new religion of a complex society does not worship the individual; it posits universal qualities and characteristics that are worshipped (Pickering 1984).

The true religion of the cult of humanity 'implies commitment to the liberty of others, to their rights and to the notion of social and economic justice' (Pickering 1984: 486). These sentiments are clearly echoed in public health, and in health promotion concerns for empowerment and social justice. The perspective discussed in chapter 3, where public health initiatives foster 'non-exploitive' communities based on equity and human rights (Lawrence and Fudge 2007) can be read as closely aligning with a vision of a cult of humanity.

Science and Religion

Durkheim believed that, with the development of modern society, science would come to play an increasingly important part in the lives of everyone. Science would encroach upon the domain previously controlled by religion. Yet religion would still be important. Durkheim seemed ambivalent on this point as he argued that science would continue to be subordinate to religion, and yet will take a critical attitude to religion. In addition religion would have to take science into account: 'Scientific thought cannot rule alone. There is, and there will always be, room in social life for a form of truth which will perhaps be expressed in a very secular way, but will nevertheless have a mythological and religious basis' (Durkheim cited in Mestrovic 1991: 82).

Yet Durkheim is an advocate of science and rationalism. Some view this as implying that Durkheim conceived of future religions as being basically rational (Pickering 1984) and that faith would be based on reason. The relation of scientific thought to religious thought for Durkheim is not simply one where science equals truth and religion equals falsity, as 'religious beliefs rest upon a specific experience whose demonstrative value is, in one sense, not one bit inferior to that of scientific experiments' (Durkheim 1915: 417). More fundamental to this is the fact that Durkheim perceives the scientific category of thought (in fact all categories of thought) as being of religious origin. For example, communal activity with its associated rites gives rise to the abstract category of time (ibid.: 440). Individuals would not develop this concept of time by themselves, but can only do so in relation to others.

Durkheim sees both religious thought and scientific thought as attempts to translate the realities of nature, humanity and society into intelligible language. They differ in that science brings in a spirit of criticism and attempts to set aside passion and subjectivity: 'Scientific thought is only a more perfect form of religious thought' (Durkheim 1915: 429). Science takes over the cognitive and intellectual functions that were previously the domain of religion. But science is always fragmentary and incomplete, and so religion will continue to fulfil a speculative function that science does not allow itself.

We can see this tension and the incomplete nature of science, and public health science, in the words of the epidemiologist Austin Bradford Hill, as noted in chapter 2: 'All scientific work is liable to be upset or modified by advancing knowledge' (cited in Pratt 2004: 231). This is the dilemma for public health – to advance beyond 'certain' knowledge and prematurely complete it in order to act. Petersen and Lupton (1996: 43) note that epidemiological researchers 'tend to be cautious about making strongly worded recommendations based on their findings' but that public health workers dispense with such caution and make strong statements about the importance of health promoting activities. Here lies a tension in public health between advocacy (with its strong component of moral regulation) and science (cautious, tentative and critical).

Science exerts a critical control over religion. Religion cannot deny what science affirms (Durkheim 1915). Yet Durkheim also states that scientific concepts that are held collectively are always in the minority. What may be true may not be believed as it does not fit in with other collective representations and, further, 'science rests upon opinion' (ibid.: 438). There is a sense of ambivalence here, and although Durkheim is a rationalist and a believer in science, he is aware of problems of science and its socially constructed aspects. For Durkheim however, both religion and science are collective representations that mark an objective truth (Hamnett 1984: 206), but Durkheim was unable to give science a position of epistemological privilege over other types of thought, including religious thought.

Durkheim also makes a point of distinguishing religion from magic, which is important when looking for manifestations of the cult of humanity in contemporary society. Magic does not create bonds that bring the magician and the clientele into a lasting community. The relationship between the magician and the client is like that between the physician and the sick person (Nisbet 1965: 83). So medicine by itself, or therapeutic interventions at an individual level, cannot constitute the new religion. Interventions at a community or population level are much more aligned with the concept of the cult of humanity. The science of social epidemiology underpinning public health policy can be seen in terms of this new religion based on reason and objective knowledge.

Public Health and Restraint

Public health has many characteristics that suggest it fills the role of religion in contemporary society. A concern for health is one thing we can share in common. We all have experiences of disease and disability throughout our lives, and a particular state of health allows individuals to participate in society. In public health, personal health is seen in relation to community health. For example, a measure of the success of national public health and social justice outcomes includes life-expectancy tables, as noted in chapter 2. Health can be seen as an individualistic pursuit; however, the notion of public health is inherently a collective representation, where individual health goals can be framed within the concept of population health.

Public health is also a buffer against anomie as it regulates individuals and limits their endless pursuit of pleasures. Health promotion campaigns, which are based on an assumption of the rational management of populations through the active intervention of individuals in making healthy choices (Fox 1998), exemplify this. Major common health promotion campaigns have included the targeting of smoking, exercise and food consumption.

The 'war' against the obesity epidemic is a most obvious manifestation of a particular public health focus on lifestyle. In England it is estimated that three-quarters of the adult population are overweight, and the economic costs are many billions of pounds a year as a consequence of heart disease, diabetes and other chronic conditions (Peckham 2007). A great deal of research effort and intervention has gone into tackling this epidemic and improving the eating and exercise habits of nations around the world. Some of this has focused on promoting behavioural change, but attention has also been paid to the obesogenic environment. Calls for constraint in eating are made and the concept of the obesogenic environment is deployed to critique the activities of multinational food manufacturing companies (Chopra and Darnton-Hill 2004). In chapter 3 it was noted that in some jurisdictions food policies have been introduced into publicly funded schools to limit unhealthy food options. Porter (2008) notes this in the U.S.A., where the Surgeon General's Office has restricted the availability of high calorie, high fat foods in schools. For many public health advocates these efforts do not go far enough, and governments are seen to have failed to tackle the root cause of obesity – 'a toxic environment created by corporate capitalist greed' (ibid.: 51). As such, the excesses of both individual behaviour and the behaviour of individual capitalist enterprises are targets for public health advocates. Public health acts to moderate these excesses.

The concept of healthy public policy illustrates the way in which public health can be used as a tool to constrain other institutional activities. The Ottawa Charter intended to make health the responsibility of policy makers in all sectors (Scriven 2007: 119). The Second International Conference on Health Promotion in Adelaide in 1998 recommended that 'healthy public policies' were 'concerned with health and equity at all levels of policy' (ibid.: 120). Specifically, as Scriven argues, a healthy public policy 'assigns high priority to tackling inequalities in health and to underprivileged and vulnerable groups', 'promotes equal access to health services' and 'recognises the link between health and social reform' (ibid.: 120). In addition healthy public policies 'are based on democratic concepts involving participation, empowerment and emancipation' (ibid.: 122).

In 1986 WHO identified five principles of healthy public policy which included that: 'economic development must seek to increase quality of life and not just gross national product' and 'health for all requires the collaboration of all policy sectors' (Scriven 2007: 123). Intersectoral action is necessary to deal with chronic disease, as the social determinants of disease lie outside the health sector. It is increasingly common to have public health positioned as an area of concern for all agencies. Parish argues that 'improving public health is therefore a multi-sectoral, multidisciplinary endeavour, requiring all sectors to play a part. Moreover, the dividend arising from better health will also be felt by all sections of society' (Parish 2007: xv).

This concept of healthy public policy is used to push for policy initiatives and developments to focus on the 'healthy citizen', drawing in government, non-government and community agencies to achieve this goal (Petersen and Lupton 1996). Health impact assessment (HIA) has been developed as a mechanism to pursue the goal of healthy public policy, where a risk assessment of the possible health impacts of policies is made so as to influence policy in a health-positive way.

Health impact assessment (HIA) may be a relatively new phrase but is not a new phenomenon. Chapters 1 and 2 showed how the appeal to health concerns to address infrastructural issues can be found in the early phase of modern public health. The expansion of towns led to fears that wet conditions would turn roads into miasma-fomenting muddy tracks, such fears provoking municipal authorities into action (Wood 2005). It was also feared that smelly and unsightly rubbish heaps would become sites of disease-carrying germs when the concept of the germ attained prominence (ibid.).

Today, HIA has been institutionalized in international organizations. The WHO promotes HIA as a means of ensuring that the health consequences of policy decisions are taken into consideration (Smith et al. 2010). A special rapporteur for the United Nations Commission on Human Rights called for health impact assessments to be used in the context of the WTO (Labonté and Schrecker 2009). Article 152 of the European Union's Amsterdam Treaty states that 'a high level of human health protection shall be ensured in the definition and implementation of all Community policies and activities' (European Centre for Health Policy 1999: 1). Underlying values in HIA include democracy and equity (ibid.). HIA involves the examination of policies and programmes to assess their potential impact on health and to suggest adjustments that will ensure a positive impact on health. A further extension of public health into policy can be seen in the concept of 'health in all policies' which aims to get all government sectors and agencies to address the determinants of health, and not simply assess the impact of policies on health. In 2007, South Australia embarked upon a process of attempting to instigate a 'health in all policies' programme (Kickbusch et al. 2008).

The influence of HIA on policy decision making is variable. There are extant examples where HIAs have led to changes to proposals, such as occurred with the Manchester Airport HIA (Quigley and Taylor 2004). Within some nation-states HIA has been embedded in public health policy (Knutsson and Linell 2010). There is, however, some pessimism over the capacity of HIA to influence policy decisions when other forms of impact assessment compete for policy influence, such as business impact assessments. In the European Union this is the case, where HIA, subsumed into social impact assessment, has been integrated into a process that includes environmental and business impact assessment (Smith et al. 2010). British American Tobacco, for example, was able to influence the European Union's impact assessment process so that its focus was on business and not on health (ibid.). Despite this, public health appears to be one of the few means of resistance to those international agencies whose activities and goals fostering free markets and capitalist enterprise can negatively impact on health and exacerbate health inequalities.

It has been argued that the social dislocation resulting from the imposition of market capitalism on traditional economic forms produces anomie (Labonté 2008). That is, the property relations under capitalism with a focus on individual title break up collective forms of ownership, and the requirement for individual consumers and mobile producers breaks up the traditional bonds of culture, and so on. The increasing break up of collective associations such as trade unions, have led, according to some, to a focus on lifestyle as a form of identity formation and compulsive morbid behaviour (ibid.). In this context public health can be seen as one form of restraint against this individualization, and a contemporary form of collective solidarity limiting the impact of anomie.

Rituals

Rituals, particular social practices that unite the community, are important features of religion and the cult of humanity. Public health rituals, which may act to encourage restraint, purify, or reinforce particular values, are increasingly prominent.

The criticism of public health for being a tool of social engineering and curbing individual freedom, although often coming from the targets of public health policies such as tobacco companies (Blackstone 2005), indicates the way in which the individual is restricted and controlled by the imperative to respect the rights of other human beings. This can be seen in many public health campaigns, such as tobacco control policy that has limited where people can smoke (Bauer et al. 2005). The notion that rituals will focus on purity can be applied to this domain of smoking, where the concept of second-hand smoke has been effectively used to separate out smokers from non-smokers in many public spaces. Other rituals deal with transgression and are central to the renewal or reconstitution of society (Ramp 2003). Media coverage of vaccines, where children adversely affected by an infectious disease are displayed as warnings to recalcitrant parents to foster conformity to vaccine schedules, reinforces the ritual of vaccination. The technology of immunization can be seen as another powerful tool in subsuming the individual to the collective will, where the concept of herd immunity is invoked to foster campaigns to increase compliance with the technology, as noted in chapter 6.

A more recently inaugurated ritual unites the globe around environmental concerns. The 'Earth Hour' event first occurred in 2007 in Sydney, when households and businesses turned lights off for one hour as a symbolic representation of concerns about climate change. In 2010, participation in 'Earth Hour' occurred across 128 countries (Earth Hour 2010). There are few real benefits in terms of climate change from such an annual event, but a ritualistic one-hour darkening unites the globe in a collective activity fostering awareness and solidarity.

Public health rituals have combined with rituals of remembrance. The 'Relay for Life' events sponsored by cancer societies, which incorporate ceremonies of remembrance alongside health promotion campaigns (McGuinness 2002), illustrate developments in this direction. Relay for Life started in 1985 when a colorectal surgeon from Tacoma, Washington, ran and walked around a track for twenty-four hours to raise money for the American Cancer Society. This has now grown into an event that has 3.5 million participants each year in the U.S. alone. Besides running and walking there are many other ritualistic features of the Relay for Life, including a Luminaria ceremony. In this ceremony candles are lit inside sand-filled bags, each one bearing the name of someone 'touched by cancer' (Relay for Life/American Cancer Society 2010). The Relay for Life has an explicit goal of unifying communities.

Rituals of restraint have progressively become internalized over time, and may no longer need public health campaigns to raise awareness or promote particular activities. In chapter 1, we encountered the increasing levels of self-restraint that occurred in relation to nineteenth-century worries over sanitation. Norbert Elias argues that society has undergone a 'civilising process' – in which we have become more restrained in our manners with a lower threshold of embarrassment (Elias 1978). The process is a result of divergent groups increasingly mixing. This internalization of social control and the development of manners relates to social density. Standards of what is normal and what is deviant become more stringent. Examples can be taken from books of manners that were written in Europe in the sixteenth century, suggesting that we should not return chewed up meat to the communal plate or wipe snot on the table cloth. This development of personal restraint is not policed by formal forces – such as the clergy, the police, the medical profession or public health advocates – but is an outcome of everyday interaction.

The following examples are used by Elias to illustrate the changes in self-restraint between contemporary and early modern times:

> There are those who teach that the boy should retain wind by compressing the belly. Yet it is not pleasing ... If it is possible to withdraw, it should be done alone. But if not, in accordance with the ancient proverb, let a cough hide the sound. (Erasmus 1530, cited in Elias 1978: 130)

> Moreover, it does not befit a modest, honourable man to prepare to relieve nature in the presence of other people ... It is far less proper to hold out the stinking thing for the other to smell, as some are wont, who even urge the other to do so, lifting the foul-smelling thing to his nostrils and saying 'I should like to know how much that stinks,' when it would be better to say, 'Because it stinks do not smell it.' (Della Casa 1558, cited in Elias 1978: 131)

The shift in social mores is clear from these quotes. To hold out faecal matter for others to assess in terms of its pungency would now be seen as such a major infraction of social rules that it would elicit the most powerful of social sanctions. There is no need for a book of manners to mention such issues today as these matters are policed and internalized in the early years of a child's development.

A more recent intervention to deal with immorality, as well as disease, was the provision of public toilets in cities. Defecation and urination in an unregulated fashion in urban spaces was increasingly seen as unacceptable, and in the mid-1800s local authorities paid more attention to dealing with this behaviour. Not only did such practices lead to the problem of such filth having to be disposed of in some way, but relieving oneself in public led to the exposure of parts of the anatomy that was increasingly perceived and prescribed as 'private' (Brunton 2002).

Laws against spitting and urinating in public were required in the past to control behaviours – but these behaviours are largely internalized now. Baldwin suggests that the same kind of internalization may occur with tobacco smoking and exhalation, where what appear to some to be draconian laws to prohibit smoking in a range of public places will become internalized in the same way as we would not now think, in the normal run of things, to urinate or defecate in the streets (Baldwin 2008).

The Collective Ritual of the Fun Run

Public health collective rituals can also be seen on a mass scale, most clearly evident in 'fun runs' (Dew and Gardner, forthcoming). In fun runs we see the development of collective rituals in which the values of society are reaffirmed. The goal of improving the health of the individual through collective effort is apparent in these very popular gatherings.

In August every year over 75,000 people gather at Sydney's Hyde Park to participate in an impressive public health collective ritual – the 14-kilometre 'city2surf' run (Astbury 2009). The collective and non-elitist nature of the fun runs can be seen in the changing nature of Sydney's city2surf run, which since its inception in 1971 as a serious race, has transformed into possibly the biggest fun run in the world, with average running times doubling as more and more amateurs participate (ibid.). In New Zealand the annual 8.4-kilometre 'Round the Bays' fun run in Auckland attracts over 70,000 participants, and the annual 13-mile Great North Run in England attracted 38,000 participants in 2005. Within these collective activities there has been increasing evidence of expressions of individuality. Many participants dress up for the occasion – Spiderman suits, medieval regalia and bright pink costumes may be witnessed. In England there are such runs as the 'funny bunny' run in Derbyshire – where people are encouraged to dress up as bunnies.

By paying fees and through sponsorship, each participant raises money for a range of charities. The ritual is also a site of contestation around public health messages. Fitness and a healthy lifestyle are projected. In 2009, a team of 1,542 was entered into the Round the Bays run by the Auckland region's district health boards, whose members were treated to vegetarian patties and salads on completion of the run. In contrast, the event's sponsors included purveyors of junk food and alcohol, and chocolate bars were given out to every participant.

But for all this, the event is one of physical activity that relates to current public health understandings of heart health. Coronary heart disease is the most common cause of death for women in the U.K. and the U.S. (Adams et al. 2008) and vies for cancer as one of the major causes of death in developed countries (New Zealand Health Information Service 2006).

In the past, rituals have been enacted to ward off epidemics of infectious diseases – the major cause of mortality up until the twentieth century. The ancient Greeks, for example, would introduce new gods to their pantheon (Nutton 2006), and in Medieval Europe conspicuous displays of wealth and fashion were banned during epidemics to appease the anger of God. The ritual scourging of flagellants in response to the Black Death in fourteenth-century Europe (Hays 2005) is well known.

In more contemporary times, new rituals have been instituted to ward off diseases of leisure and plenty, the diseases of wealth as opposed to the diseases of poverty. Sometimes these rituals are individually enacted, such as the lone jogger pounding the streets; sometimes there is communal participation, such as working out in the gym or team sports, and occasionally a collective gathering, as with fun runs and marathons.

Rituals like the fun run not only provide a collective symbolic response to concerns about contemporary disease, but also unite society in a communal activity, a social practice, that asserts particular values of the society. These activities can be read as promoting particular moral forces, reinforcing particular forms of social order. The moral imperative to be a responsible citizen requires care of the heart, and attention to the risks of an early death. We regularly encounter persuasive public health campaigns to get us out and about and active. The regular fun run is a collective ritual that provides a meaningful statement about healthy hearts and population health – the heart itself at the centre of humanity.

The Mayor of Sydney identified many of the communal values that are being reinforced through collective rituals such as fun runs: 'Sydney Mayor Clover Moore termed yesterday's run "a celebration of our beautiful, outward-looking city and the lively and diverse people within it, our sense of community, our love of the outdoors and healthy living"' (Ansari 2009).

The fun run reinforces notions of how lucky we (Australians in this instance) are to live in such a country. Nationhood is reinforced, but not at the expense of some particular 'out' groups. Diversity is embraced – runners of all kinds of ability can participate, and if you cannot run, you walk. A sense of community is manifest as such a vast horde of people – a city of people – enact the same ritual, negotiate the same course, achieve the same goals and experience a sense of connectedness with others in the event, promoting communal values of health. The valorization of the outdoors and hardiness to counterbalance the soft life of office workers and couch potatoes is clearly made. Notions of discipline, self-control and self-efficacy are reinforced. Anyone can participate, if they are willing to get up and give it a go. But at the same time there are winners, there are elite runners, there is a meritocracy at play. The collective activity of fun runs embraces both mediocrity and excellence. Just as these supposed opposites are embraced, individuality is not excluded from communal participation. Costumes might be worn to signify difference from others, but all take the same route and have the same goal of getting to the finish line. Altruism, in opposition to egoism, is most evident in the money raised for charity – with the Sydney city2surf raising $AUS2 million.

As noted, science plays an important part in this new religion. Science determines references to 'objective knowledge' about social and personal worlds; the new religion's faith, therefore, is based on reason. Fun runs for health and the quest for a healthy heart are embedded in a long history of developments in medicine and science. In order to connect up in a meaningful way the heart, health and physical activity, many elements needed to come together. It required the particular understandings of anatomy, pathology, statistics and a range of technological developments. It required William Harvey's vivisections on animals in the 1600s to develop a model of the circulation of the blood. The heart had to be conceived of as a muscle that needs exercise. It required the development of classification codes for diseases, so that heart conditions could be distinguished from respiratory, gastric and other conditions. It required the concept of the 'normal distribution', developed in statistics, so that populations of the idle could be compared to populations of the active. And, it required stethoscopes and electrocardiograms (ECGs) so that something occurring inside the body could be heard or seen from the outside.

Out of this intricate interplay of concepts and technologies arises a particular picture of the heart health of the population, along with the identification of risk factors for premature death from heart disease and recommendations on how to prevent it. This is the territory of the cult of humanity, where individual health is seen in relation to the population and health takes on a universal quality, where disparities in health between groups can be demonstrated, and where the negative impact of fast food and indolence on the population can be articulated. Public health provides a moral force to temper anomic and egoistic drives to consumption and sloth. The collective fun runs are astounding events saturated with meaning that are a contemporary manifestation of collective worship and self-responsibility.

Esurient and Absolutist Public Health

It has been argued here that public health acts as a particular moral force in contemporary society. But public health is also esurient; it has a voracious appetite for consuming the social world in its efforts to make all that is around it a part of itself. We can see a number of dimensions of this esurience. One manifestation of public health esurience is seen in our most basic activities, such as walking, being shaped in the form of public health. The fun runs noted above are extraordinary events, but walking is an everyday event. Public health discourses on walking have drenched this mundane activity in moral overtones. Walking is advocated as an activity that can have a positive impact on public health in many ways. It can improve one's individual health by exercising muscles, improving the heart rate and helping to overcome the negative health consequences of a sedentary life. It can also contribute to the reduction of environmental pollution of the immediate environment, reducing particulates in the surrounding air that could negatively impact on respiratory conditions. Additionally, it can help save the planet. Sustainable cities where citizens participate increasingly in active transport (walking, running, cycling) and less in transport relying on the petrochemical industry or other forms of energy that might negatively impact on the environment, will help to combat global warming and contribute to saving lives on the planet (Green 2009).

In order to achieve some of these gains, walking is constructed in a particular way. Walking must be of a certain speed and a certain frequency (Green 2009). In addition, certain types of walking put one at health risk, for example, in deprived urban areas where walking children are more likely to be injured in traffic accidents. As traffic has increased, safe spaces for children have been reduced, which differentially impacts upon poorer neighbourhoods (Freund and Martin 2008). In other situations, where the deprivation of going without is chosen and not unavoidable, walking is valorized.

Tramping across the countryside without the usual accoutrements of urban living is seen as an accomplishment, but one that is usually available to the middle class (Green 2009). In this situation, deprivation itself has a moral value as it is associated with choice and leisure (ibid.). That is, walking as an experience and as a symbolic activity varies greatly according to the social, historical and political factors at play. It can be an empowering activity for the middle classes, but a disempowering one for the working classes and the materially deprived. So the middle classes can obtain moral value from walking, whereas for many others it is a burden forced upon them because of lack of access to resources. This everyday activity is presented within public health discourses as 'unproblematically healthy' (ibid.).

Population health perspectives have also moulded clinical practice, which was discussed in detail in chapter 4. The development of prioritization tools for elective services has shifted clinicians from a patient advocacy to a population health perspective. Tools used to prioritize patient conditions have also been used to show patients why they might not be able to access publicly funded services. Clinicians have reported that this has muted individual protests about not getting access to these services, as patients see that there are others in a worse position than they are (Dew et al. 2005a). As such, public health perspectives on justice and fairness have permeated individual clinical consultations.

Efforts to bring about policy change are in the domain of public health (Sanders 2009). However, the advocacy role of public health can tend to absolutism. One interesting manifestation of the tendency towards absolutism can be seen in calls for universities to prohibit researchers from associating with tobacco companies (Cohen 2001). From a public health critique of tobacco companies, this is one small weapon against the tobacco companies' odious impact on human health. Academic research can give credibility to tobacco companies. Tobacco companies could show how altruistic they are by supporting a variety of research, and such altruism is deceptive and should not be allowed. Academics should not associate with such a deadly industry. The arguments that can be made to support such a prohibition are many and varied. But universities are one of the few sites of intellectual independence and academic freedom, which can include a right, or even a responsibility, to test conventional wisdom. Public health esurience has deprived academics of that right in many universities across the globe. In this instance, the advocacy function has subsumed the academic function of public health, where limitations are placed on the activities of scientists in the name of public health. The moral regulation of capitalism has overwhelmed the academic freedom and critical conscience role of universities.

Public health is anything but a static institution. It adapts to new situations. Public health responses to population health are connected to the diversifying impacts of global movements and also the homogenizing effect of technological developments, norms and manners. When we consider what it is we have in common, our humanity, we also have a complex issue related to genetic composition, human physiology, social organization and the natural environment that plays out in public health. Technological developments allowing for genetic testing and screening limit the range of what we perceive to be the norms of humanity. As Bauman puts it: 'whatever is defined today as bodily deformity or mere abnormality may well be criminalized, while the list of deformities and abnormalities will be growing unstoppably as the mapping of chromosomes, and expanding the inventory of available tinkering practices proceeds at an accelerating pace' (1995: 179). There is the potential for increasingly individualized information about our risks of disease and propensities. These technologies, in a Foucauldian vein, enhance surveillance and the potential for interventions (Bunton and Petersen 2008).

Public health can be called upon to support the development of a fit and healthy population for the purposes of war, and for the purposes of work. In either arena, once prepared through public health interventions, the population can be exposed to conditions hazardous to life. For all its extensive reach, public health can still fail to meet the needs of the most vulnerable groups in society. The eugenics and racial hygiene movements in the first half of the twentieth century warn us of the part that public health can play, wittingly or unwittingly, in rituals of purification that have terrible consequences for some population groups.

Discussion

An uncritical acceptance of Durkheimian concepts, which have received sustained critique (see Hirst 1975 for a critique of his epistemological assumptions and logic), is not claimed here, but it is argued that drawing on Durkheimian concepts sheds light on the function of public health in contemporary society. A case has been presented for considering the activity of public health in all its manifestations as a candidate for Durkheim's cult of humanity. Such a view provides insight into the dual advocacy and academic functions of public health, the tension between individual choice and constraint, and the buffering role that public health takes in relation to other societal institutions. With public health, the basic functions of humanity such as drinking, eating and moving are integrated into a system of meaning related to the collective good. Public health appears to be a prime candidate for fulfilling the role of religion in a society based on organic solidarity.

In his view of radicalized modernity, Giddens places much faith in social movements as providing an impetus to transformation with coordinated political engagement as necessary on both a global and a local level. Chapter 2 demonstrated the way in which public health can indeed engage at both levels. Giddens' vision does not encompass the suggestion being made here – that an advocacy movement ambiguously placed between science and the state provides an opportunity for transformation. Having transformational potential does not imply liberation. For example, the issue of freedom of thought in public health discourse appears to be tightly constrained. Pickering argued that freedom of thought would be an important element of the cult of humanity, but the possibility of unconstrained thought does not align well with Durkheimian concerns over anomie. Regulation is a requirement to balance opposing moral forces. To a limited extent, freedom of thought may exist for those who are involved in the science of public health. The science maintains a critical function, and although perhaps limited, the self-critical functions of the scientific enterprise open up the possibility for dissenting views and debate. But this would be less the case for public health advocates and for the population as a whole. Individual views about such things as immunization and second-hand smoke need to be tightly constrained so as not to undermine public campaigns.

The new public health has been viewed as both an extension of regulatory forces and a force for emancipation (Jones 2001). The rhetorical focus on equity, empowerment and community mobilization in healthy public policy and the new public health signal the emancipatory potential (ibid.). Baggott (2000) argues that the collectivist positioning of public health 'includes ameliorating the health damaging consequences of individualism and tackling the socio-economic causes of ill health generated by capitalism (ibid: 3). In other words, public health tempers both the egoistic tendencies of individualism and restrains the anomic tendencies generated by capitalism. Baggott goes on to suggest that 'the appeal to resist the market on the grounds of health is a powerful one' (ibid.: 3) . But from a Durkheimian perspective, rather than focus on the notion of emancipation, the core features of these developments in public health are the countervailing forces to unrestrained bureaucracy and markets. As Donald Light has argued, countervailing powers in health care, which include the state and the medical profession, cannot be in an ideal state of balance. One power may dominate at any one time, and 'such dominance produces its own pathologies by carrying its goals to extremes' (Light 1997: 107). As such, public health itself is not a force of emancipation, but an institutional means to provide some balance to the absolutist tendencies in social spheres outside of the health domain. Public health then acts as a moral force in many spheres: at the individual level in relation to the regulation of individual behaviours that restrain the excesses of consumerism, at an institutional level in relation to such mechanisms as HIA, and, more tentatively, at an international level in relation to covenants like the FCTC. As Labonté and Schrecker argue, health could be taken as a shared value that can define a global community (Labonté and Schrecker 2009).

Public health can be positioned as a buffer against both individualism and capitalism. With this understanding, public health researchers and advocates have a clearer view of their objectives, and the potential confusion between politics and science can be explained. The role of public health in moral regulation can be seen as a contemporary response to the limits of traditional religions, but as such public health will always be in tension with the individualistic tendencies at the foundation of the human condition, represented in Durkheim's use of the concept *homo duplex*. Another role that public health has the potential to play is as a mediator between the abstract understandings of experts and the complex, messy, everyday life of social practices. The understandings of experts, or those with authority to set standards and develop protocols, do not always reflect the lived reality of those who are expected to conform to those standards. This issue has been illustrated with examples from workers in factories, farmers on farms and health professionals in consultation rooms. Public health researchers and advocates who are closer to the communities of interest have opportunities to bridge this gap between idealized models and actual practices.

The argument put forward here also suggests some potentially testable hypotheses and research areas. If public health plays a part in the moral regulation of society then it can be suggested that different population groups may be more open to public health responses than others. If we take the view that the cult of humanity will take most hold in the more socially differentiated and individualized groups (Hill 1987), then we would expect these people to be most responsive to public health messages. The moral regulation of public health would temper the potential for excessive consumption and 'endless desiring'. As such, the urbanized middle classes, who have a history of social and geographical mobility, would be the most likely candidates to conform to public health messages related to smoking, alcohol and food consumption, and exercise. Other groups who are already morally regulated may not be so susceptible. For example, adolescents who have a strong sense of identity with peers may not be so responsive to public health messages. Groups that function along the lines of mechanical solidarity, with low levels of social differentiation and traditional forms of authority, may not be so susceptible. We can consider here some tightly knit working-class groups, like the larrikin subculture discussed in chapter 3.

Drawing on Durkheimian insights we can consider the role of public health in ways that have not been emphasized in the extant literature. From a Durkheimian perspective, public health research can be seen as an instrument determining the pathological and the normal by comparisons of death rates between populations along such dimensions as class, gender and ethnicity, comparisons of health services utilization between populations, and so on. As such, public health explicitly links Durkheim's concern for justice with his concepts of the normal and the pathological. The descriptive science of social epidemiology then forms the foundation of a morality.

There is a distinctively different use of the concept of the normal in Foucauldian and Durkheimian analyses, where the notion of normalization is itself seen in pathological terms within a Foucauldian framing. In addition, Foucauldian-style analyses focus on the genealogy and dispersion of discourses. There is a tendency to see resistance to such discourses as an individual response. From a Foucauldian perspective, resistance to the normalizing process appears as a response to the struggle for one's own identity that can then be linked to collective struggles (McNay 1992). Embedded within networks of power, the imagery tends to be of individual efforts to resist. Conflict perspective explorations of public health tend to position the institution as a problem (in league with capital) or as a solution (a focus on social determinants undermining individualizing tendencies that foster reliance on the free market). An exploration of public health in relation to the cult of humanity suggests a different focus. Public health is an institution that performs a moral regulatory function in contemporary society, and therefore as an institution is in opposition or conflict with other institutions performing different regulatory functions or fostering individualism.

Resistance, from this perspective, is not conceptualized at an individual level, but at a collective level. However, resistance itself may not be the best term; rather a tempering of different regulatory regimes may better describe interactions between institutions. From this standpoint, power can be absolutist when any particular regulatory regime dominates, and that power can historically be seen as waxing and waning for different institutions – including bureaucracies, the market, public health and academia. Public health should not simply be seen as a negative or positive force. Unrestrained public health is absolutist, but public health itself can restrict the negative impact of other institutions and restrain egoistic and anomic tendencies in contemporary society.

Bibliography

Adbusters, n.d. Journal of the Mental Environment. Retrieved 28 January 2010 from https://www.adbusters.org/gallery/spoofads.

Adkins, L. 2002. 'Risk, Sexuality and Economy', *British Journal of Sociology* 53(1), 19–40.

Aira, M., J. Kauhanen, P. Larivaara and P. Rautio. 2003. 'Factors Influencing Inquiry about Patients' Alcohol Consumption by Primary Care Physicians: Qualitative Semi-structured Interview Study', *Family Practice* 20(3), 270–75.

Ajwani, S., T. Blakely, B. Robson, M. Tobias and M. Bonne. 2003. *Decades of Disparity: Ethnic Mortality Trends in New Zealand 1980–1999*. Wellington: New Zealand Ministry of Health.

Allender, S., D. Colquhuon and P. Kelly. 2006. 'Competing Discourses of Workplace Health', *Health* 10(1), 75–93.

Amos, A. 2007. 'From Self-regulation to Legislation: The Social Impact of Public Health Action on Smoking', in A. Scriven and S. Garman (eds), *Public Health: Social Context and Action*. Maidenhead: Open University Press, pp. 193–205.

Ansari, K. 2009. 'World's Largest Fun Run', *Mid Day*. Retrieved 8 December 2009 from http://www.mid-day.com/news/2009/aug/100809-Bondi-beach-London-New-York-marathons.htm.

Apollonio, D.E. and R.E. Malone. 2009. 'Turning Negative into Positive: Public Health Mass Media Campaigns and Negative Advertising', *Health Education Research* 24(3), 483–95.

Armstrong, D. 1983. *Political Anatomy of the Body: Medical Knowledge in Britain in the Twentieth Century*. Cambridge: Cambridge University Press.

——— 1995. 'The Rise of Surveillance Medicine', *Sociology of Health and Illness* 17, 393–404.

Asbury, L.D., F.I. Wong, S.M. Price and M.J. Nolin. 2008. 'The VERB™ Campaign: Applying a Branding Strategy in Public Health', *American Journal of Preventive Medicine* 34(6), S183–S187.

Ashmore, M., M. Mulkay and T. Pinch. 1989. *Health and Efficiency: A Sociology of Health Economics*. Milton Keynes: Open University Press.

Astbury, S. 2009. World's Biggest Race is Just a Fun Run. *Monsters and Critics*. Retrieved 4 December 2009 from http://www.monstersandcritics.com/news/

asiapacific/features/article_1494739.php/World-s-biggest-race-is-just-a-fun-run-News-Feature.
Atkinson, W. 2007. 'Beck, Individualization and the Death of Class: A Critique', *British Journal of Sociology* 58(3), 349–66.
Baggott, R. 2000. *Public Health: Policy and Politics*. Basingstoke: Palgrave.
Baldwin, P. 2008. 'Can There be a Democratic Public Health? Fighting AIDS in the Industrialized World', in S. Gross Solomon, L. Murard and P. Zylberman (eds), *Shifting Boundaries of Public Health: Europe in the Twentieth Century*. Rochester: University of Rochester Press, pp. 23–44.
Ballantyne, C. 2007. 'Strange but True: Antibacterial Products May Do More Harm Than Good', *Scientific American* 296(6), http://www.scientific american.com/article.cfm?id=strange-but-true-antibacterial-products-may-do-more-harm-than-good.
Banerji, D. 1990. 'Crash of the Immunization Program: Consequences of a Totalitarian Approach', *International Journal of Health Services* 20, 501–10.
Barnes, B. 1995. *The Elements of Social Theory*. Princeton: Princeton University Press.
Barrett, G., J. Naidoo and J. Orme. 2007. 'Capacity and Capability in Public Health', in J. Orme, J. Powell, P. Taylor and M. Grey (eds), *Public Health for the 21st Century: New Perspectives on Policy, Participation and Practice*. Maidenhead: Open University Press, pp. 83–97.
Barrow, L. 2002. 'In the Beginning was the Lymph: The Hollowing of Stational Vaccination in England and Wales, 1840–98', in S. Sturdy (ed.), *Medicine, Health and the Public Sphere in Britain, 1600–2000*. London and New York: Routledge, pp. 205–23.
Barta, T. 2005. 'Mr Darwin's Shooters: On Natural Selection and the Naturalizing of Genocide', *Patterns of Prejudice* 39(2), 116–17.
Bauer, J., A. Hyland, Q. Li, C. Steger and K.M. Cummings. 2005. 'A Longitudinal Assessment of Smoke-free Worksite Policies on Tobacco Use', *American Journal of Public Health* 95(6), 1024–29.
Bauld, L. and M. Mackenzie. 2007. 'Health Action Zones: Multi-agency Partnerships to Improve Health', in A. Scriven and S. Garman (eds), *Public Health: Social Context and Action*. Maidenhead: McGraw Hill/Open University Press, pp. 131–43.
Bauman, Z. 1995. *Life in Fragments: Essays in Postmodern Morality*. Oxford (U.K.) and Cambridge, MA: Blackwell.
——— 2000. *Liquid Modernity*. Cambridge: Polity Press.
Bazeley, P. 1989. 'Public and Private Immunization Services: A Comparison of Costs', *Community Health Studies* 13, 336–40.
Beaglehole, R. 1992. 'Prospects for Public Health in New Zealand', *New Zealand Medical Journal* 105(927), 29–31.
Beaglehole, R. and R. Bonita. 1997. *Public Health at the Crossroads: Achievements and Prospects*. Cambridge: Cambridge University Press.
Beck, U. 1992. *Risk Society: Towards a New Modernity*. London: Sage.
——— 1995. *Ecological Politics in an Age of Risk*. Cambridge: Polity Press.

Belgrave, M. 1985. '"Medical Men" and "Lady Doctors": The Making of a New Zealand Profession, 1867–1941', Ph.D. dissertation. Wellington: Victoria University of Wellington.

Berg, M. 1997. *Rationalizing Medical Work: Decision-support Techniques and Medical Practices*. Cambridge, MA: MIT Press.

Berg, M. and P. Harterink. 2004. 'Embodying the Patient: Records and Practices in Early 20th Century U.S. Medical Practice', *Body and Society* 10(2), 13–41.

Bingham, A. 1992. *National Task Group on Site Contamination: Task Brief 5: Dioxin Regulations and Guidelines*. Wellington: Ministry for the Environment.

Birkmeyer, J.D. and H.G. Welch. 1993. 'Rationing Surgery: Rules or Constraints?', *Surgery* 113(5), 491–97.

Birn, A.E. 1999. 'Skirting the Issue: Women and International Health in Historical Perspective', *American Journal of Public Health* 89(3), 399–407.

Blackstone, B. 2005. 'U.S. Anti-smoking Plan is Criticized', *Wall Street Journal*, 9 June, B2.

Blakely, T., M. Tobias, B. Robson, S. Ajwani, M. Bonné and A. Woodward. 2005. 'Widening Ethnic Mortality Disparities in New Zealand 1981–99', *Social Science and Medicine* 61(10), 2233–51.

Bloom, S.W. 2002. *The World as Scalpel: A History of Medical Sociology*. New York: Oxford University Press.

Bloomfield, A., P. Didsbury, N. Sharpe and R. Jackson. 1999. 'Accessing and Using Evidence in Practice: New Zealand Opportunities and Resources', *New Zealand Public Health Report* 6(7), 49–52.

Borowy, I. 2008. 'Manoeuvring for Space: International Health Work of the League of Nations during World War II', in S. Gross Solomon, L. Murard and P. Zylberman (eds), *Shifting Boundaries of Public Health: Europe in the Twentieth Century*. Rochester: University of Rochester Press, pp. 87–113.

Boseley, S. 2010. 'Andrew Wakefield Struck Off Register by General Medical Council', *The Guardian*, 24 May 2010.

Bridgstock, M. 1982. 'A Sociological Approach to Fraud in Science', *Australian and New Zealand Journal of Sociology* 18(3), 364–83.

Britan, G.M. 1981. *Bureaucracy and Innovation: An Ethnography of Policy Change*. Beverly Hills: Sage.

Brody, H., M. Rip, P. Vinten-Johansen, N. Paneth and S. Rachman. 2000. 'Map-making and Myth-making in Broad Street: The London Cholera Epidemic, 1854', *The Lancet* 356, 64–68.

Brown, E.R. 1994. *Rockefeller Medicine Men: Medicine and Capitalism in America*. Berkeley: University of California Press.

Brown, P. 1989. 'Popular Epidemiology: Community Response to Toxic Waste-induced Disease in Woburn, Massachusetts', in P. Brown (ed.), *Perspectives in Medical Sociology*. Belmont: Wadsworth.

Brulle, R. and D. Pellow. 2006. 'Environmental Justice: Human Health and Environmental Inequalities', *Annual Review of Public Health* 27, 103–24.

Brunner, E. and M. Marmot. 1999. 'Social Organization, Stress and Health', in M. Marmot and R. Wilkinson (eds), *Social Determinants of Health*. Oxford: Oxford University Press, pp. 17–43.

Brunton, D. 2002. 'Policy, Powers and Practice: The Public Response to Public Health in the Scottish City', in S. Sturdy (ed.), *Medicine, Health and the Public Sphere in Britain, 1600–2000*. London and New York: Routledge, pp. 171–88.

Bryder, L. 1982. 'Lessons of the 1918 Influenza Epidemic in Auckland', *New Zealand Journal of History* 16(2), 97–121.

Bu, L. and E. Fee. 2008. 'John B. Grant: International Statesman of Public Health', *American Journal of Public Health* 98(4), 628–29.

Bunton, R. and A. Petersen. 2008. 'Genetics, Governance and Ethics', in J. Green and R. Labonté (eds), *Critical Perspectives in Public Health*. Abingdon and New York: Routledge, pp. 219–27.

Carroll, P. 2010. 'Capturing Realities of Informal Housing in Aotearoa/New Zealand', Ph.D. Thesis, *Public Health*. Wellington: University of Otago.

Chaitow, L. 1987. *Vaccination and Immunization: Dangers, Delusions and Alternatives*. Saffron Walden: C.W. Daniel.

Cheng, M. 2007. 'Officials Say Drug Caused Nigeria Polio', *The Washington Post*, 5 October.

Chopra, M. and I. Darnton-Hill. 2004. 'Tobacco and Obesity Epidemics: Not So Different After All', *British Medical Journal* 328(7455), 1558.

Clark, W.C. 1980. 'Witches, Floods, and Wonder Drugs: Historical Perspectives on Risk Management', in R.C. Schwing and W.A. Albers (eds), *Societal Risk Assessment: How Safe is Safe Enough?* New York and London: Plenum Press, pp. 287–318.

Coburn, D. 1999. 'Phases of Capitalism, Welfare States, Medical Dominance, and Health Care in Ontario', *International Journal of Health Services* 29(4), 833–51.

Coburn, D., S. Rappolt and I. Bourgeault. 1997. 'Decline vs Retention of Medical Power through Restratification: An Examination of the Ontario Case', *Sociology of Health and Illness* 19, 1–22.

Cockburn, A. 1996. 'Alexander Cockburn's America: It Seems Black Children May Be Victims of the Medical Establishment', *New Statesmen*, p. 25.

Cohen, J. 2001. 'Universities and Tobacco Money', *British Medical Journal* 323, 1–2.

Cohen, P. 1995. 'Doctors Cheat Because They Know What's Best', *New Scientist*, 2008, 10.

Cohet, C., S. Cheng, C. MacDonald, M. Baker, S. Foliaki, N. Huntingdon, J. Douwes and N. Pearce. 2004. 'Infections, Medication Use, and the Prevalence of Symptoms of Asthma, Rhinitis and Eczema in Childhood', *Journal of Epidemiology and Community Health* 58, 852–57.

Collin, J. and K. Lee. 2007. 'Globalization and Public Health Policy', in A. Scriven and S. Garman (eds), *Public Health: Social Context and Action*. Maidenhead: McGraw Hill/Open University Press, pp. 105–15.

Commission for the Environment 1985. *The ICI Fire: A Report to the Minister for the Environment*, Wellington, New Zealand.

Conner-Spady, B., G. Arnett, J. McGurran and T. Noseworthy. 2004. 'Prioritization of Patients on Scheduled Waiting Lists: Validation of a Scoring System for Hip and Knee Arthroplasty', *Canadian Journal of Surgery* 47(1), 39–46.

Copp, N. and A. Zanella. 1992. *Discovery, Innovation and Risk: Case Studies in Science and Technology*. Cambridge, MA: MIT Press.

Costello, A., M. Abbas, A. Allen, S. Ball, S. Bell, R. Bellamy, S. Friel, N. Groce, A. Johnson, M. Kett, M. Lee, C. Levy, M. Maslin, D. McCoy, B. McGuire, H. Montgomery, D. Napier, C. Pagel, J. Patel, J. Antonio, P. de Oliveira, N. Redclift, H. Rees, D. Rogger, J. Scott, J. Stephenson, J. Twigg, J. Wolff and C. Patterson. 2009. 'Managing the Health Effects of Climate Change', *The Lancet* 373(9676), 1693–733.

Coulter, I. 2004. 'Integration and Paradigm Clash: The Practical Difficulties of Integrative Medicine', in P. Tovey, G. Easthope and J. Adams (eds), *The Mainstreaming of Complementary and Alternative Medicine: Studies in Social Context*. London and New York: Routledge, pp. 103–22.

CSDH 2008. *Closing the Gap in a Generation: Health Equity through Action on the Social Determinants of Health. Final Report of the Commission on Social Determinants of Health*. Geneva: World Health Organization.

Cumming, J. 1994. 'Core Services and Priority-setting: The New Zealand Experience', *Health Policy* 29(1–2), 41–60.

Curtis, S. and A. Taket. 1996. *Health and Societies: Changing Perspectives*. London: Arnold.

Dahlgren, G. and M. Whitehead. 1991. *Policies and Strategies to Promote Social Equity in Health*. Stockholm: Institute of Futures Studies.

Dale, P., J. Greenlees and J. Melling. 2007. 'The Kiss of Death or a Flight of Fancy? Workers' Health and the Campaign to Regulate Shuttle Kissing in the British Cotton Industry, c.1900–1952', *Social History* 32(1), 54–75.

Das, D., M. Baker, K. Venugopal and S. McAllister. 2006. 'Why the Tuberculosis Incidence Rate is Not Falling in New Zealand', *New Zealand Medical Journal* 119(1243).

Datta, J. and A. Kessell. 2010. 'Unlinked Anonymous Blood Testing for Public Health Purposes: An Ethical Dilemma?', in S. Peckham and A. Hann (eds), *Public Health Ethics and Practice*. Bristol: The Policy Press, pp. 101–15.

Davis, P. 1981. *Health and Health Care in New Zealand*. Auckland: Longman Paul.

Day, A. 2008. 'Child Immunisation: Reactions and Responses to New Zealand Government Policy 1920–1990', Ph.D. dissertation. Auckland: The University of Auckland.

Daykin, N. 1999. 'Introduction: Critical Perspectives on Health and Work', in N. Daykin and L. Doyal (eds), *Health and Work: Critical Perspectives*. Basingstoke: Macmillan Press, pp. 1–20.

Deaton, A. 2007. *Global Patterns of Income and Health: Facts, Interpretations and Policies*. Helsinki: UNU World Institute for Development Economics Research.

Dembe, A. 1998. 'The Medical Detection of Simulated Occupational Injuries: A Historical and Social Analysis', *International Journal of Health Services* 28(2), 227–39.

Devlin, N., T. Ashton and J. Cumming. 1999. 'Rationing Health Care: How Should the HFA Proceed?', *New Zealand Medical Journal* 112(1097), 369–70.

Dew, K. 1999a. 'Epidemics, Panic and Power: Representations of Measles and Measles Vaccines', *Health* 3(4), 379–98.

——— 1999b. 'National Identity and Controversy: New Zealand's Clean Green Image and Pentachlorophenol', *Health and Place* 5(1), 45–57.

——— 2002. 'Accident Insurance, Sickness and Science: New Zealand's No-fault System', *International Journal of Health Services* 32(1), 163–78.

——— 2003. 'Neo-European Risk and Biosecurity: The Release of Rabbit Viruses in Australasia', *New Zealand Sociology* 18(1), 202–24.

——— 2007. 'Public Health and the Cult of Humanity: A Neglected Durkheimian Concept', *Sociology of Health and Illness* 29(1), 100–14.

Dew, K. and P. Carroll. 2007. 'Public Health and CAM Perspectives: An Exploration of Overlap, Contrast and Dissonance', in J. Adams (ed.), *Researching Complementary and Alternative Medicine*. Abingdon and New York: Routledge, pp. 117–32.

Dew, K., J. Cumming, D. McLeod, S. Morgan, E. McKinlay, A. Dowell and T. Love. 2005a. 'Explicit Rationing of Elective Services: Implementing the New Zealand Reforms', *Health Policy* 74(1), 1–12.

Dew, K. and J. Gardner, forthcoming. 'Rituals of the Heart', in P. Howland and I. Day (eds), *Ritual: Aotearoa New Zealand*. Wellington: CANZ in association with Steele Roberts Publishers.

Dew, K., V. Keefe and K. Small. 2005b. '"Choosing" to Work When Sick: Workplace Presenteeism', *Social Science and Medicine* 60(10), 2273–82.

Dew, K., M. Stubbe, L. Macdonald, A. Dowell and E. Plumridge. 2010. 'The (Non) Use of Prioritisation Protocols by Surgeons', *Sociology of Health and Illness* 32(4), 545–62.

Dew, K. and K. Taupo. 2009. 'The Moral Regulation of the Workplace: Presenteeism and Public Health', *Sociology of Health and Illness* 31(7), 994–1010.

Dreyfus, H. and P. Rabinow. 1982. *Michel Foucault: Beyond Structuralism and Hermeneutics*. Brighton: Harvester Press.

Dubos, R. 1965. *Man Adapting*. New Haven: Yale University Press.

Durbach, N. 2000. 'They Might as Well Brand Us: Working Class Resistance to Compulsory Vaccination in Victorian England', *Social History of Medicine* 13(1), 45–62.

Durkheim, E. 1915. *The Elementary Forms of the Religious Life: A Study in Religious Sociology*. London: George Allen and Unwin.

——— 1957. *Professional Ethics and Civic Morals*. London: Routledge.

Dwyer, T. 1991. *Life and Death at Work: Industrial Accidents as a Case of Socially Produced Error*. New York: Plenum Press.

Earth Hour 2010. Earth Hour Global Site. Retrieved 7 June 2010 from http://www.earthhour.org/Homepage.aspx?intro=no.

Eberhart-Phillips, J. 1999. *Plagues on Our Doorstep: The Threat of Infectious Disease in New Zealand.* Auckland: Tandem Press.

Ebi, K., S. Kovats and B. Menne. 2005. 'An Approach for Assessing Human Health Vulnerability and Public Health Interventions to Adapt to Climate Change', *Environmental Health Perspectives* 114(12), 1930–34.

Elias, N. 1978. *The Civilizing Process.* New York: Urizen Books.

Elias, S., D. Bandaranayake, I. Edwards and W. Glass. 1990. *The Health Consequences of the ICI Fire: Report to the Minister of Health on the Health of Firefighters in the Fire at the ICI Riverview Store, Mount Wellington, Auckland, 21 December 1984.* Wellington: Department of Health.

Elliott, A. 2002. 'Beck's Sociology of Risk: A Critical Assessment', *Sociology* 36(2), 293–315.

Ellis, R. and D. Whittington. 1993. *Quality Assurance in Health Care: A Handbook.* London: Edward Arnold.

European Centre for Health Policy 1999. *Health Impact Assessment: Main Concepts and Suggested Approach.* Gothenburg Consensus Paper, Brussels.

Evans, D. 2007. 'New Directions in Tackling Inequalities in Health', in J. Orme, J. Powell, P. Taylor and M. Grey (eds), *Public Health for the 21st Century: New Perspectives on Policy, Participation and Practice.* Maidenhead: Open University Press, pp. 155–69.

Feingold, E. 1998. 'Public Health Versus Civil Liberties', *Public Health Reports* 113(4), 334–35.

Feiring Williams, J. 1928. *Healthful Living: Based on the Essentials of Physiology for High-school Pupils.* New York: The Macmillan Company.

Feyerabend, P. 1987. *Against Method.* London: Verso.

Fielding, J. 2009. 'Commentary: Public Health and Health Care Quality Assurance—Strange Bedfellows?', *Milbank Quarterly* 87(3), 581–84.

Fleming, P. 2007. 'Workplace as Settings for Public Health Development', in A. Scriven and S. Garman (eds), *Public Health: Social Context and Action.* Maidenhead: McGraw Hill/Open University Press, pp. 166–79.

Foege, W.H. 1997. 'Public Health and Preventive Medicine', *Journal of the American Medical Association* 278, 1894–95.

Forman, J. 2008. 'Health Inequalities and Need Associated with Rare Diseases', in K. Dew and A. Matheson (eds), *Understanding Health Inequalities in Aotearoa New Zealand.* Dunedin: Otago University Press, pp. 119–29.

Foster, J.B. 1999. 'Marx's Theory of Metabolic Rift: Classical Foundations of Environmental Sociology', *American Journal of Sociology* 105(2), 366–405.

Foucault, M. 1978. *The History of Sexuality: An Introduction.* London: Allen Lane.

——— 1988. 'The Political Technology of Individuals', in L. Martin, H. Gutman and P.H. Hutton (eds), *Technologies of the Self: A Seminar With Michel Foucault.* Amherst: University of Massachusetts Press.

Fox, N. 1993. *Postmodernism, Sociology and Health*. Buckingham: Open University Press.

——— 1998. 'Postmodernism and Health', in A. Peterson and C. Waddell (eds), *Health Matters: A Sociology of Illness, Prevention and Care*. St Leonards: Allen and Unwin, pp. 9–22.

Freidson, E. 1986. 'The Medical Profession in Transition', in L.H. Aiken and D. Mechanic (eds), *Applications of Social Science to Clinical Medicine and Health Policy*. New Brunswick: Rutgers University Press, pp. 63–79.

——— 1994. *Professionalism Reborn: Theory, Prophecy and Policy*. Chicago: The University of Chicago Press.

Freund, P. and G. Martin. 2008. 'Moving Bodies: Injury, Dis-ease and the Social Organisation of Space', in J. Green and R. Labonté (eds), *Critical Perspectives in Public Health*. London and New York: Routledge, pp. 228–35.

Fudge, C. 2007. 'Implementing Sustainable Futures in Cities', in J. Orme, J. Powell, P. Taylor and M. Grey (eds), *Public Health for the 21st Century: New Perspectives on Policy, Participation and Practice*. Maidenhead: Open University Press, pp. 185–203.

Gerhardt, U. 1989. *Ideas about Illness: An Intellectual and Political History of Medical Sociology*. Basingstoke: Macmillan.

Giddens, A. 1990. *The Consequences of Modernity*. Stanford: Stanford University Press.

——— 1991. 'Structuration Theory: Past, Present and Future', in C. Bryant and D. Jary (eds), *Theory of Structuration: A Critical Appreciation of Giddens*. London: Routledge, pp. 201–21.

Gidley, B. 2007. 'Sure Start: An Upstream Approach to Reducing Health Inequalities', in A. Scriven and S. Garman (eds), *Public Health: Social Context and Action*. Maidenhead: McGraw Hill/Open University Press, pp. 144–53.

Gilbert, N. and M. Mulkay. 1984. *Opening Pandora's Box: A Sociological Analysis of Scientists' Discourse*. Cambridge: Cambridge University Press.

Gilbert, P. 2002. 'Producing the Public: Public Medicine in Private Spaces', in S. Sturdy (ed.), *Medicine, Health and the Public Sphere in Britain, 1600–2000*. London: Routledge, pp. 43–59.

Gilchrist, A. 2007. 'Community Development and Networking for Health', in J. Orme, J. Powell, P. Taylor and M. Grey (eds), *Public Health for the 21st Century: New Perspectives on Policy, Participation and Practice*. Maidenhead: Open University Press, pp. 135–52.

Gillespie, J.A. 2008. 'Europe, America, and the Space of International Health', in S. Gross Solomon, L. Murard and P. Zylberman (eds), *Shifting Boundaries of Public Health: Europe in the Twentieth Century*. Rochester: University of Rochester Press, pp. 114–37.

Glantz, S. and E. Balbach. 2000. *Tobacco War: Inside the California Battles*. Berkeley: University of California Press.

Glasgow, R., T. Vogt and S. Boles. 1999. 'Evaluating the Public Health Impact of Health Promotion Interventions: The RE-AIM Framework', *American Journal of Public Health* 89, 1322–27.

Goffman, E. 1963. *Stigma: Notes on the Management of Spoiled Identity*. Englewood Cliffs: Prentice-Hall.

——— 2006. 'On Face-work', in G. Massey (ed.), *Readings for Sociology*. New York: W.W. Norton and Company, pp. 105–14.

Gorman, D. and E. Dryson. 1998. 'Diagnosis of Chemical Poisoning: Report of a Working Party Established by the Australasian Faculty of Occupational Medicine, Royal Australian College of Physicians, Auckland, 9 May 1997', *New Zealand Medical Journal* 111(1059), 34–37.

Gray, B., C. Brunton and P. Barnett. 2006. 'The Law Reform (Epidemic Preparedness) Bill: A Proper Response to the Pandemic Threat?' *New Zealand Medical Journal* 119(1240), 1–8.

Gray, S. 2007. 'The Contribution of Health Services to Public Health', in J. Orme, J. Powell, P. Taylor and M. Grey (eds), *Public Health for the 21st Century: New Perspectives on Policy, Participation and Practice*. Maidenhead: Open University Press, pp. 118–34.

Green, J. 2008. 'Introduction to Part IV', in J. Green and R. Labonté (eds), *Critical Perspectives in Public Health*. Abingdon and New York: Routledge, pp. 204–12.

——— 2009. '"Walk This Way": Public Health and the Social Organization of Walking', *Social Theory and Health* 7(1), 20–38.

Green, J. and R. Labonté. 2008a. 'Introduction: From Critique to Engagement. Why Critical Public Health Matters', in J. Green and R. Labonté (eds), *Critical Perspectives in Public Health*. Abingdon and New York: Routledge, pp. 1–11.

——— 2008b. 'Preface: Public Health as Social Activism. A Slightly Abashed Hagiography', in J. Green and R. Labonté (eds), *Critical Perspectives in Public Health*. Abingdon and New York: Routledge, pp. xiii–xiv.

Grey, M., M. Studden and J. Sarangi. 2007. 'Protecting the Public's Health', in J. Orme, J. Powell, P. Taylor and M. Grey (eds), *Public Health for the 21st Century: New Perspectives on Policy, Participation and Practice*. Maidenhead: Open University Press, pp. 223–50.

Gross Solomon, S., L. Murard and P. Zylberman. 2008. 'Introduction', in S. Gross Solomon, L. Murard and P. Zylberman (eds), *Shifting Boundaries of Public Health: Europe in the Twentieth Century*. Rochester: University of Rochester Press, pp. 1–20.

Haas, B. 1994. 'Problematic Characteristics of the Public Deliberation on Core Health Services', *New Zealand Sociology* 9(1), 36–58.

Hacking, I. 1990. *The Taming of Chance*. Cambridge: Cambridge University Press.

Haines, A., P. Wilkinson, C. Tonne and I. Roberts. 2009. 'Aligning Climate Change and Public Health Policies', *The Lancet* 374(9707), 2035–37.

Hales, S., V. Baker, K. Dew, L. Moata'ane, J. Martin, T. Rochford, D. Slaney and A. Woodward. 2004. *Assessment of the Potential Health Impacts of the 'Painted Apple Moth' Aerial Spraying Programme, Auckland*. Wellington: New Zealand Ministry of Health.

Hall, W. 1989. 'The Logic of Controversy: The Case of Agent Orange in Australia', *Social Science and Medicine* 29(4), 537–44.

Halliday, S. 2007. *The Great Filth: The War Against Disease in Victorian England*. Chalford, Stroud: Sutton Publishing.

Hamilton, M., P. Corwin, S. Gower and S. Rogers. 2004. 'Why Do Parents Choose Not to Immunise Their Children', *New Zealand Medical Journal* 117(1189), 768.

Hamlin, C. 2002. 'Public Sphere to Public Health: The Transformation of "Nuisance"', in S. Sturdy (ed.), *Medicine, Health and the Public Sphere in Britain, 1600–2000*. London and New York: Routledge, pp. 189–204.

Hamlin, C. and S. Sheard. 1998. 'Revolutions in Public Health: 1848 and 1998?', *British Medical Journal* 317(7158), 587–91.

Hammond, P. 1974. 'Religious Pluralism and Durkheim's Integration Thesis', in A. Eister (ed.), *Changing Perspectives in the Scientific Study of Religion*. New York: John Wiley and Sons, pp. 115–42.

Hamnett, I. 1984. 'Durkheim and the Study of Religion', in S. Fenton (ed.), *Durkheim and Modern Sociology*. Cambridge: Cambridge University Press, pp. 202–18.

Hannigan, J.A. 1995. *Environmental Sociology*. London and New York: Routledge.

Hansen, A. 1991. 'The Media and the Social Construction of the Environment', *Media, Culture and Society* 13, 443–58.

Hansen, E. and G. Easthope. 2007. *Lifestyle in Medicine*. London and New York: Routledge.

Hardy, A. 2001. *Health and Medicine in Britain since 1860*. Houndmills: Palgrave.

Hays, J.N. 2005. *Epidemics and Pandemics: Their Impacts on Human History*. Santa Barbara: ABC-CLIO.

Heath, C. 1992. 'The Delivery and Reception of Diagnosis in the General-Practice Consultation', in P. Drew and J. Heritage (eds), *Talk at Work: Interaction in Institutional Settings*. Cambridge: Cambridge University Press, pp. 235–67.

Heath, C. and P. Luff. 2000. *Technology in Action*. Cambridge: Cambridge University Press.

Heller, J. 2008. *The Vaccine Narrative*. Nashville: Vanderbilt University Press.

Hersey, J.C., J. Niederdeppe, S.W. Ng, P. Mowery, M. Farrelly and P. Messeri. 2005. 'How State Counter-industry Campaigns Help Prime Perceptions of Tobacco Industry Practices to Promote Reductions in Youth Smoking', *Tobacco Control* 14, 377–83.

Herzfeld, M. 1992. *The Social Production of Indifference: Exploring the Symbolic Roots of Western Bureaucracy*. Chicago: University of Chicago Press.

Higginbotham, N., G. Albrecht and S. Freeman. 2001. 'Heart Disease in Transdisciplinary Perspective', in N. Higginbotham, G. Albrecht and L. Connor (eds), *Health Social Science: A Transdisciplinary and Complexity Perspective*. Melbourne: Oxford University Press, pp. 93–114.

Higgs, P. and I.R. Jones. 2001. 'Finite Resources and Infinite Demand: Public Participation in Health Care Rationing', in G. Scambler (ed.), *Habermas, Critical Theory and Health*. London and New York: Routledge, pp. 143–62.

Hill, M. 1987. 'The Cult of Humanity and the Secret Religion of the Educated Classes', *New Zealand Sociology* 2, 112–27.

Hirst, P. 1975. *Durkheim, Bernard and Epistemology*. London and Boston: Routledge and Kegan Paul.

Hobson-West, P. 2007. '"Trusting Blindly Can Be the Biggest Risk of All": Organised Resistance to Childhood Vaccination in the UK', *Sociology of Health and Illness* 29(2), 198–215.

Holt, E. 2010. 'Debate Over Health Effects of Chernobyl Re-ignited', *The Lancet* 375(9724), 1424–25.

Host, J. 1998. *Victorian Labour History: Experience, Identity and the Politics of Representation*. London and New York: Routledge.

Howell, P. 2000. 'A Private Contagious Diseases Act: Prostitution and Public Space in Victorian Cambridge', *Journal of Historical Geography* 26(3), 376–402.

Hunter, D. 2007a. 'Public Health Policy', in J. Orme, J. Powell, P. Taylor and M. Grey (eds), *Public Health for the 21st Century: New Perspectives on Policy, Participation and Practice*. Maidenhead: Open University Press, pp. 24–41.

——— 2007b. 'Public Health: Historical Context and Current Agenda', in A. Scriven and S. Garman (eds), *Public Health: Social Context and Action*. Maidenhead: McGraw Hill/Open University Press, pp. 8–19.

Hyde, P. 1999. 'Health Promotion and Health Technology', in P. Davis and K. Dew (eds), *Health and Society in Aotearoa New Zealand*. Auckland: Oxford University Press, pp. 255–69.

——— 2000. 'Science Friction: Cervical Cancer and the Contesting of Medical Beliefs', *Sociology of Health and Illness* 22, 217–34.

Inhorn, M.C. and K.L. Whittle. 2001. 'Feminism Meets the "New" Epidemiologies: Toward an Appraisal of Antifeminist Biases in Epidemiological Research on Women's Health', *Social Science and Medicine* 53(5), 553–67.

Irwin, A., A. Dale and D. Smith. 1996. 'Science and Hell's Kitchen: The Local Understanding of Hazard Issues', in A. Irwin and B. Wynne (eds), *Misunderstanding Science? The Public Reconstruction of Science and Technology*. Cambridge: Cambridge University Press, pp. 47–64.

Izuretia, H.S., P.M. Strebel and P.A. Blake. 1997. 'Postlicensure Effectiveness of Varicella Vaccine during an Outbreak in a Child Care Center', *Journal of the American Medical Association* 278, 1495–99.

Jacobson, P., J. Wasserman and J. Anderson. 1997. 'Historical Overview of Tobacco Legislation and Regulation', *Journal of Social Issues* 53(1), 75–95.

James, L. 1994. *The Rise and Fall of the British Empire*. London: Abacus.

Jeffreys, T. 1998. *Your Health at Risk: What Doctors and the Government Aren't Telling You*. Auckland: Howling at the Moon Publishing.

Johnston, R. 2006. *The Radical Middle Class: Populist Democracy and the Question of Capitalism in Progressive Era Portland, Oregon*. Princeton: Princeton University Press.

Jones, I. 2001. 'Health Care Decision Making and the Politics of Health', in G. Scambler (ed.), *Critical Theory and Health*. London: Routledge, pp. 68–85.

Jost, T.S. 1992. 'Recent Developments in Medical Quality Assurance and Audit', in R. Dingwall and P. Fenn (eds), *Quality and Regulation in Health Care: International Experiences*. London: Routledge, pp. 69–88.

Kawachi, I., R. Wilkinson and B. Kennedy. 1999. 'Introduction', in I. Kawachi, R. Wilkinson and B. Kennedy (eds), *The Society and Population Health Reader: Volume 1 Income Inequality and Health*. New York: The New Press, pp. xi–xxxiv.

Keenan, B. 2007. *Leptospirosis: Reducing the Impact on New Zealand Workplaces*. Wellington: Department of Labour.

Kendall, S. 1998. 'Introduction', in S. Kendall (ed.), *Health and Empowerment: Research and Practice*. London: Arnold, pp. 1–7.

Kickbusch, I., W. McCann and T. Sherbon. 2008. 'Adelaide Revisited: From Health Public Policy to Health in All Policies', *Health Promotion International* 23(1), 1–4.

King, M. 2007. 'Mass Media, Lifestyle and Public Health', in A. Scriven and S. Garman (eds), *Public Health: Social Context and Action*. Maidenhead: McGraw Hill/Open University Press, pp. 95–104.

Klein, R., P. Day and S. Redmayne. 1996. *Managing Scarcity: Priority Setting and Rationing in the National Health Service*. Buckingham: Open University Press.

Knight, J. 1999. 'Models of Health', in J. Germov (ed.), *Second Opinion: An Introduction to Health Sociology*. Melbourne: Oxford University Press, pp. 136–55.

Knutsson, I. and A. Linell. 2010. 'Health Impact Assessment Developments in Sweden', *Scandinavian Journal of Public Health* 38(2), 115–20.

Kohler-Moran, S., S. Wolff and J. Green. 1995. 'Workers' Compensation and Occupational Stress: Gaining Control', in L. Murphy, J. Hurrell, S. Sauter and G.P. Keita (eds), *Job Stress Interventions*. Washington, DC: American Psychological Association, pp. 355–68.

Koplan, J.P., A.R. Hinman, R.L. Parker, Y.L. Gong and M.D. Yang. 1985. 'The Barefoot Doctor: Shanghai County Revisited', *American Journal of Public Health* 75(7), 768–70.

Krieger, N. 2001. 'Theories for Social Epidemiology in the 21st Century: An Ecosocial Perspective', *International Journal of Epidemiology* 30, 668–77.

Labonté, R. 2008. 'Introduction to Part III', in J. Green and R. Labonté (eds), *Critical Perspectives in Public Health*. Abingdon and New York: Routledge, pp. 136–49.

Labonté, R. and T. Schrecker. 2009. 'Rights, Redistribution and Regulation', in R. Labonté, T. Schrecker, C. Packer and V. Runnels (eds), *Globalization and Health: Pathways, Evidence and Policy*. New York and London: Routledge, pp. 317–33.

Labonté, R. and R. Torgerson. 2008. 'Interrogating Globalisation, Health and Development: Towards a Comprehensive Framework for Research, Policy and Political Action', in J. Green and R. Labonté (eds), *Critical Perspectives in Public Health*. Abingdon and New York: Routledge, pp. 162–79.

Lambert, L. and E. Wenzel. 2008. 'Medicine Keepers: Issues in Indigenous Health', in J. Green and R. Labonté (eds), *Critical Perspectives in Public Health*. Abingdon and New York: Routledge, pp. 180–91.

Lange, R. 1999. *May the People Live: A History of Māori Health Development 1900–1920*. Auckland: Auckland University Press.

Larkin, M. 2008. 'Globalisation and Health', in J. Green and R. Labonté (eds), *Critical Perspectives in Public Health*. Abingdon and New York: Routledge, pp. 151–61.

Latour, B. 1987. *Science in Action*. Cambridge, MA: Harvard University Press.

——— 1994. *The Pasteurization of France*. London: Harvard University Press.

Lawlor, D., S. Keen and R. Neal. 2000. 'Can General Practitioners Influence the Nation's Health through a Population Approach to Provision of Lifestyle Advice?', *British Journal of General Practice* 50, 455–59.

Lawrence, P. and C. Tibbitts. 1951. 'Recent Long-term Morbidity Studies in Hagerstown, MD', *American Journal of Public Health* 41(8), 101–7.

Lawrence, R. and C. Fudge. 2007. 'Healthy Cities: Key Principles for Professional Practice', in A. Scriven and S. Garman (eds), *Public Health: Social Context and Action*. Maidenhead: McGraw Hill/Open University Press, pp. 180–92.

Lee, J.S. 1996. 'Adult Immunization Priorities in the United States', *The Milbank Quarterly* 74, 285–307.

Leith, V.M.S. 2007. 'Consent and Nothing but Consent? The Organ Retention Scandal', *Sociology of Health and Illness* 29(7), 1023–42.

Li, J., E. Mattes, F. Stanley, A. McMurray and C. Hertzman. 2009. 'Social Determinants of Child Health and Well-being', *Health Sociology Review* 18(1), 3–11.

Light, D.W. 1997. 'The Rhetorics and Realities of Community Health Care: The Limits of Countervailing Powers to Meet the Health Care Needs of the Twenty-first Century', *Journal of Health Politics Policy and Law* 22(1), 105–45.

Lindfors, P. and L. Raevaara. 2005. 'Discussing Patients' Drinking and Eating Habits in Medical and Homeopathic Consultations', *Communication and Medicine* 2(2), 137–49.

Lippman, S. and E. Hawk. 2009. 'Cancer Prevention: From 1727 to Milestones of the Past 100 Years', *Cancer Research* 69(13), 5269–84.

Lohr, K., K. Eleazer and J. Mauskopf. 1998. 'Health Policy Issues and Applications for Evidence-based Medicine and Clinical Practice Guidelines', *Health Policy* 46, 1–19.

Lomas, J. and A.P. Contandriopoulos. 1994. 'Regulating Medicine: Towards Harmony in Public- and Self-regulation', in R.G. Evans, M.L. Barer and T.R. Marmor (eds), *Why are Some People Healthy and Others Not? The Determinants of Health of Populations*. New York: Aldine De Gruyter, pp. 253–83.

Luckin, B. 2002. 'The Shaping of a Public Environmental Sphere in Late Nineteenth-century London', in S. Sturdy (ed.), *Medicine, Health and the Public Sphere in Britain, 1600–2000*. London and New York: Routledge, pp. 224–40.

Lukes, S. 1973. *Emile Durkheim: His Life and Work*. Harmondsworth: Penguin.

Lupton, D. 1994. *Medicine as Culture: Disease and the Body in Western Societies*. London: Sage.

MacDonald, T. 1998. *Rethinking Health Promotion: A Global Approach*. London: Routledge.

Maclean, F.S. 1964. *Challenge for Health – A History of Public Health in New Zealand*. Wellington: Government Printer.

Major, G. n.d. *Lifestyle Talk and Advice in Clinical Consultations: Working Paper*. Wellington: University of Otago.

Manning, P. 1992. *Erving Goffman and Modern Sociology*. Stanford: Stanford University Press.

Marmor, T.R., M.L. Barer and R.G. Evans. 1994. 'The Determinants of a Population's Health: What Can be Done to Improve a Democratic Nation's Health Status?', in R.G. Evans, M.L. Barer and T.R. Marmor (eds), *Why are Some People Healthy and Others Not? The Determinants of Health of Populations*. New York: Aldine De Gruyter, pp. 217–30.

Marmot, M., S. Friedl, R. Bell, T. Houweling and S. Taylor. 2008. 'Closing the Gain in a Generation: Health Equity through Action on the Social Determinants of Health', *The Lancet* 372(9650), 1661–69.

Martin, B. 1991. *Scientific Knowledge in Controversy: The Social Dynamics of the Fluoridation Debate*. Albany: State University of New York Press.

——— 1996. 'Sticking a Needle into Science: The Case of Polio Vaccines and the Origin of AIDS', *Social Studies of Science* 26(2), 245–76.

Matheson, A., K. Dew and J. Cumming. 2009. 'Complexity, Evaluation and the Effectiveness of Community-based Interventions to Reduce Health Inequalities', *Health Promotion Journal of Australia* 20(3), 221–26.

Matthews, J.R. 1995. *Quantification and the Quest for Medical Certainty*. Princeton: Princeton University Press.

Maynard, A. 1995. 'Distributing Health Care Rationing and the Role of the Physician in the United Kingdom National Health Service', in A. Grubb and M.J. Mehlman (eds), *Justice and Health Care: Comparative Perspectives*. Chichester: John Wiley and Sons, pp. 305–21.

——— 1996. 'Rationing Health Care', *British Medical Journal* 313(7071), 1499.

McAvoy, B. 2000. 'A Scandal of Inaction: How to Help GPs Implement Evidence-based Health Promotion', *British Journal of General Practice* 50, 180–81.

McAvoy, B., E. Kaner, C. Lock, N. Heather and E. Gilvarry. 1999. 'Our Healthier Nation: Are General Practitioners Willing and Able to Deliver? A Survey of Attitudes to and Involvement in Health Promotion and Lifestyle Counselling', *British Journal of General Practice* 49, 187–90.

McClean, S. 2007. 'Globalization and Health', in J. Orme, J. Powell, P. Taylor and M. Grey (eds), *Public Health for the 21st Century: New Perspectives on Policy, Participation and Practice*. Maidenhead: Open University Press, pp. 204–22.

McGrath, J. 1989. 'The Incidence and Notification of Measles in Australia', *Community Health Studies* 13, 156–60.

McGuinness, R. 2002. 'American Cancer Society Signature Activity: Relay for Life', *International Journal of Cancer* 100, suppl. 13, 312–13.

McKeown, T. 1979. *The Role of Medicine*. Oxford: Basil Blackwell.

McKinlay, E., L. Plumridge, L. McBain, D. McLeod, S. Pullon and S. Brown. 2005. '"What Sort of Health Promotion Are You Talking About?": A Discourse Analysis of the Talk of General Practitioners', *Social Science and Medicine* 60, 1099–106.

McLeod, D., S. Morgan, E. McKinlay, K. Dew, J. Cumming, A. Dowell and T. Love. 2004. 'Use of, and Attitudes to, Clinical Priority Assessment Criteria in Elective Surgery in New Zealand', *Journal of Health Services Research and Policy* 9(2), 91–99.

McNay, L. 1992. *Foucault and Feminism*. Cambridge: Polity Press.

Mechanic, D. 1997. 'Muddling Through Elegantly: Finding the Proper Balance in Rationing', *Health Affairs* 16, 83–92.

Mellor, P. 2004. 'Religion, Culture and Society in the "Information Age"', *Sociology of Religion* 65, 357–71.

Merton, R.K. 1973. *The Sociology of Science: Theoretical and Empirical Investigations*. Chicago and London: The University of Chicago Press.

Mestrovic, S. 1988. *Emile Durkheim and the Reformation of Sociology*. Totowa: Rowman and Littlefield.

——— 1991. *The Coming Fin De Siecle: An Application of Durkheim's Sociology to Modernity and Postmodernism*. London: Routledge.

Mooney, G. 2008. 'British Public Health and the Problem of Local Demographic Structure', in S. Gross Solomon, L. Murard and P. Zylberman (eds), *Shifting Boundaries of Public Health: Europe in the Twentieth Century*. Rochester: University of Rochester Press, pp. 205–27.

Morgan, A. and J. Popay. 2007. 'Community Participation for Health: Reducing Health Inequalities and Building Social Capital', in A. Scriven and S. Garman (eds), *Public Health: Social Context and Action*. Maidenhead: McGraw Hill/Open University Press, pp. 154–65.

Murard, L. 2008. 'Designs Within Disorder: International Conferences on Rural Health Care and the Art of the Local, 1931–39', in S. Gross Solomon, L. Murard and P. Zylberman (eds), *Shifting Boundaries of Public Health: Europe in the Twentieth Century*. Rochester: University of Rochester Press, pp. 141–74.

Muraskin, W. 1995. 'Bucking the Health Establishment: Alexander Milne and the Fight for a New Zealand Hepatitis B Immunization Program', *Social Science and Medicine* 41, 211–25.

Murphy, R. 1994. *Rationality and Nature: A Sociological Inquiry into a Changing Relationship*. Boulder, CO: Westview Press.

National Task Group 1992. *Report of the National Task Group Investigating Site Contamination from the Use of Timber Treatment Chemicals*. Wellington: Ministry for the Environment.

Natrass, N. 2008. 'AIDS and the Scientific Governance of Medicine in Post-apartheid South Africa', *African Affairs* 107(427), 157–76.

Nelkin, D. and L. Tancredi. 1994. *Dangerous Diagnostics: The Social Power of Biological Information*. Chicago: University of Chicago Press.

Nelson, R. and J. Moser. 2008. 'Controversy Surrounds Gardasil', *American Journal of Nursing* 108(7), 17.

Nettleton, S. 1985. 'Protecting a Vulnerable Margin: Towards an Analysis of How the Mouth Came to be Separated from the Body', *Sociology of Health and Illness* 10, 156–69.

New, S.J. and M.L. Senior. 1991. '"I Don't Believe in Needles": Qualitative Aspects of a Study into the Uptake of Infant Immunisation in Two English Health Authorities', *Social Science and Medicine* 33, 509–18.

New Zealand Health Information Service 2006. *Mortality and Demographic Data 2002 and 2003*. Wellington: New Zealand Ministry of Health.

New Zealand Ministry of Health 2004. *Report on the Effects of the Painted Apple Moth Spray Programme*. Wellington. New Zealand Ministry of Health.

Nisbet, R. 1965. *Emile Durkheim*. Englewood Cliffs: Prentice Hall.

Nord, P. 1994. 'The Welfare State in France', *French Historical Studies* 18(3), 821–38.

Nutton, V. 2006. 'The Rise of Medicine', in R. Porter (ed.), *The Cambridge History of Medicine*. Cambridge: Cambridge University Press, pp. 46–70.

Oppenheimer, G.M. 2005. 'Becoming the Framingham Study 1947–1950', *American Journal of Public Health* 95(4), 602–10.

Orme, J., J. Powell, P. Taylor and M. Grey. 2007a. 'Introduction', in J. Orme, J. Powell, P. Taylor and M. Grey (eds), *Public Health for the 21st Century: New Perspectives on Policy, Participation and Practice*. Maidenhead: Open University Press, pp. 1–3.

——— 2007b. 'Mapping Public Health', in J. Orme, J. Powell, P. Taylor and M. Grey (eds), *Public Health for the 21st Century: New Perspectives on Policy, Participation and Practice*. Maidenhead: Open University Press, pp. 7–23.

Osborne, T. 1997. 'Of Health and Statecraft', in A. Petersen and R. Bunton (eds), *Foucault: Health and Medicine*. London: Routledge, pp. 173–88.

Ozonoff, D. and L.I. Boden. 1987. 'Truth and Consequences: Health Agency Responses to Environmental Health Problems', *Science, Technology and Human Values* 12(3/4), 70–77.

Parish, R. 2007. 'Foreword', in A. Scriven and S. Garman (eds), *Public Health: Social Context and Action*. Maidenhead: Open University Press/McGraw Hill, pp. xv–xvi.

Pearse, I.H. and L.H. Crocker. 1947. *The Peckham Experiment: A Study in the Living Structure of Society*. London: George Allen and Unwin.

Peckham, S. 2007. 'Partnership Working for Public Health', in J. Orme, J. Powell, P. Taylor and M. Grey (eds), *Public Health for the 21st Century: New Perspectives on Policy, Participation and Practice*. Maidenhead: Open University Press, pp. 63–82.

Peckham, S. and A. Hann. 2010. 'Introduction: Why Public Health Ethics?', in S. Peckham and A. Hann (eds), *Public Health Ethics and Practice*. Bristol: The Policy Press, pp. 1–14.

Petersen, A. and D. Lupton. 1996. *The New Public Health: Health and Self in the Age of Risk*. St Leonards, NSW: Allen and Unwin.

Petryna, A. 2007. 'Clinical Trials Offshored: On Private Sector Science and Public Health', *BioSocieties* 2, 21–40.

Phillimore, P. and S. Moffatt. 1999. 'Narratives of Insecurity in Teesside: Environmental Politics and Health Risk', in J. Vail, J. Wheelock and M. Hill (eds), *Insecure Times: Living with Insecurity in Contemporary Society*. London: Routledge, pp. 137–53.

Phillips, T. 2009. 'Uncertainty and Contestation in the Medico-legal Field: An Ethnography of Dispute over the Legitimacy of Multiple Chemical Sensitivities', Ph.D. dissertation. Perth: University of Western Australia.

——— 2010. 'Debating the Legitimacy of a Contested Environmental Illness: A Case Study of Multiple Chemical Sensitivities', *Sociology of Health and Illness* 32(7), 1026–40.

Pickering, W. 1984. *Durkheim's Sociology of Religion: Themes and Theories*. London: Routledge and Kegan Paul.

Pierce, J. 1989. 'International Comparisons of Trends in Cigarette Smoking Prevalence', *American Journal of Public Health* 79(2), 152–57.

Pike, J. and D. Colquhoun. 2009. 'The Relationship between Policy and Place: The Role of School Meals in Addressing Health Inequalities', *Health Sociology Review* 18(1), 50–60.

Polanyi, M., T. McIntosh and A. Kosny. 2008. 'Understanding and Improving the Health of Workers in the New Economy: A Call for a Participatory Dialogue-based Approach to Work-health Research', in J. Green and R. Labonté (eds), *Critical Perspectives in Public Health*. Abingdon and New York: Routledge, pp. 123–33.

Popper, K. 1963. *Conjectures and Refutations*. London: Routledge and Kegan Paul.

——— 1972. *The Logic of Scientific Discovery*. London: Hutchinson.

Porter, D. 2008. 'The Social Contract of Health in the Twentieth and Twenty First Centuries: Individuals, Corporations and the State', in S. Gross Solomon, L. Murard and P. Zylberman (eds), *Shifting Boundaries of Public Health: Europe in the Twentieth Century*. Rochester: University of Rochester Press, pp. 45–60.

Porter, R. 2006a. 'Hospitals and Surgery', in R. Porter (ed.), *The Cambridge History of Medicine*. Cambridge: Cambridge University Press, pp. 176–210.

——— 2006b. 'Medical Science', in R. Porter (ed.), *The Cambridge History of Medicine*. Cambridge: Cambridge University Press, pp. 136–75.

Porter, T. 1995. *Trust in Numbers: The Pursuit of Objectivity in Science and Public Life*. Princeton: Princeton University Press.

Pratt, A. 2004. 'Scientific Controversies: Dissent and Debate', in K. Dew and R. Fitzgerald (eds), *Challenging Science: Issues for New Zealand Society in the 21st Century*. Palmerston North: Dunmore Press, pp. 223–39.

Puliyel, J.M. and Y. Madhavi. 2008. 'Vaccines: Policy for Public Good or Private Profit', *Indian Journal of Medical Research* 127(1), 1–3.

Quigley, R. and L. Taylor. 2004. 'Evaluating Health Impact Assessment', *Public Health* 118(8), 544–52.

Ramp, W. 2003. 'Religion and the Dualism of the Social Condition in Durkheim and Bataille', *Economy and Society* 32, 119–40.

Rappolt, S. 1997. 'Clinical Guidelines and the Fate of Medical Autonomy in Ontario', *Social Science and Medicine* 44(7), 977–87.

Rawls, A.W. 1990. 'Emergent Sociality: A Dialectic of Commitment and Order', *Symbolic Interaction* 13(1), 63–82.

Razzell, C. and P. Spence. 2005. 'Social Capital and the History of Mortality in Britain', *International Journal of Epidemiology* 34, 477–78.

Reid, P. 1999. 'Te Pupiri i te Ao o te Tangata Whenua', in P. Davis and K. Dew (eds), *Health and Society in Aotearoa New Zealand*. Auckland: Oxford University Press, pp. 51–62.

Relay for Life/American Cancer Society 2010. What is Relay for Life? Retrieved 2 June 2010 from http://www.relayforlife.org/relay/whatisrelay.

Reuters 1997. 'Orphans Used as Medical Guinea Pigs', *The Evening Post*, 11 June, p. 9.

Rhoades, E. 2003. 'The Health Status of American Indian and Alaska Native Males', *American Journal of Public Health* 93, 774–78.

Robinson, J.C. 1991. *Toil and Toxics: Workplace Struggles and Political Strategies for Occupational Health*. Berkeley: University of California Press.

Robson, B. 2008. 'What is Driving the Disparities?', in K. Dew and A. Matheson (eds), *Understanding Health Inequalities in Aotearoa New Zealand*. Dunedin: Otago University Press, pp. 19–31.

Rogers, A. and D. Pilgrim. 1995. 'This Risk of Resistance: Perspectives on the Mass Childhood Immunisation Programmes', in J. Gabe (ed.), *Medicine, Health and Risk: Sociological Approaches*. Oxford: Basil Blackwell, pp. 73–90.

Rose, G. 1991. *Compulsory Vaccination: A Statement of Concern from the Health Care Reform Group*. Australia: Health Care Reform Group.

Rosen, G. 1993. *A History of Public Health* (expanded edition). Baltimore: Johns Hopkins University Press.

Rosenberg, C.E. 1986. 'Disease and Social Order in America: Perceptions and Expectations', *The Milbank Quarterly* 64 (supplement 1), 34–55.

Rosenthal, M. 1995. *The Incompetent Doctor: Behind Closed Doors*. Buckingham: Open University Press.

Ryan, A. 2005. 'Sociological Perspectives on Health and Illness', in K. Dew and P. Davis (eds), *Health and Society in Aotearoa, New Zealand* (2nd edition). Melbourne: Oxford University Press, pp. 4–20.

Sackett, D. 2002. 'The Arrogance of Preventative Medicine', *Canadian Medical Association Journal* 167(4), 363–64.

Saltman, R.B. 1994. 'Patient Choice and Patient Empowerment in Northern European Health Systems: A Conceptual Framework', *International Journal of Health Services* 24(2), 201–29.

Sanders, D. 2009. 'Globalization, Social Determinants and the Struggle for Health', in R. Labonté, T. Schrecker, C. Packer and V. Runnels (eds), *Globalization and Health: Pathways, Evidence and Policy*. New York and London: Routledge, pp. 334–40.

Sandiford, P. 2009. 'Getting Back the Missing Men of Aotearoa: Declining Gender Inequality in NZ Life Expectancy', *Journal of Primary Health Care* 1(4), 270–77.

Sapp, J. 1990. *Where the Truth Lies: Franz Moewus and the Origins of Molecular Biology*. Cambridge: Cambridge University Press.

Scally, G. 2007. 'Sustainable Development and Public Health: Arm in Arm', in J. Orme, J. Powell, P. Taylor and M. Grey (eds), *Public Health for the 21st Century: New Perspectives on Policy, Participation and Practice*. Maidenhead: Open University Press, pp. 322–29.

Scambler, G. and A. Scambler. 1998. 'Women Sex Workers, Health Promotion and HIV', in S. Kendall (ed.), *Health and Empowerment: Research and Practice*. London: Arnold, pp. 112–25.

Scambler, G. and S. Scambler. 2007. 'Social Patterning of Health Behaviours', in A. Scriven and S. Garman (eds), *Public Health: Social Context and Action*. Maidenhead: McGraw Hill/Open University Press, pp. 34–47.

Schleiermacher, S. 2008. 'Contested Spaces: Models of Public Health in Occupied Germany', in S. Gross Solomon, L. Murard and P. Zylberman (eds), *Shifting Boundaries of Public Health: Europe in the Twentieth Century*. Rochester: University of Rochester Press, pp. 175–204.

Scott, J.C. 1998. *Seeing Like a State: How Certain Schemes to Improve the Human Condition Have Failed*. New Haven and London: Yale University Press.

Scott, W. 1988. 'Competing Paradigms in the Assessment of Latent Disorders: The Case of Agent Orange', *Social Problems* 35(2), 145–61.

Scriven, A. 2007. 'Health Public Policies: Rhetoric or Reality?', in A. Scriven and S. Garman (eds), *Public Health: Social Context and Action*. Maidenhead: McGraw Hill/Open University Press, pp. 119–30.

Seale, C. 1993. 'The Consumer Voice', in B. Davey and J. Popay (eds), *Dilemmas in Health Care*. Buckingham: Open University Press, pp. 64–80.

Seedhouse, D. 1995. 'The Way Around Health Economics' Dead End', *Health Care Analysis* 3, 205–20.

Shaffer, E., J. Brenner and T. Houston. 2005. 'International Trade Agreements: A Threat to Tobacco Control', *Tobacco Control* 14 (Supplement II), ii19–ii25.

Shaw, M., D. Dorling, R. Mitchell and G.D. Smith. 2005. 'Labour's "Black Report" Moment?', *British Medical Journal* 331(7516), 575–75.

Simmons, D. and P. Scott. 1998. 'Does the "Thunderbirds Syndrome" Still Exist?', *New Zealand Medical Journal* 11(1078), 456–58.

Singleton, V. 2005. 'The Promise of Public Health: Vulnerable Policy and Lazy Citizens', *Environment and Planning D, Society and Space* 23, 771–86.

Slapper, G. and S. Tombs. 1999. *Corporate Crime*. Harlow: Pearson Education.

Smart, B. 1985. *Michel Foucault*. Chichester: Ellis Horwood.

——— 1996. 'Postmodern Social Theory', in B.S. Turner (ed.), *The Blackwell Companion to Social Theory*. Oxford: Blackwell, pp. 396–428.

Smith, K.E., G. Fooks, J. Collin, H. Weishaar and A.B. Gilmore. 2010. 'Is the Increasing Use of Policy Impact Assessment in Europe Likely to Undermine Efforts to Achieve Healthy Public Policy', *Journal of Epidemiology and Community Health* 64(6), 478–87.

Smith, R. 1991. 'Where is the Wisdom?', *British Medical Journal* 393, 798–99.

Smith, V. 2007. *Clean: A History of Personal Hygiene and Purity*. Oxford: Oxford University Press.

Smyth, R.M.D., J.J. Kirkham, A. Jacoby, D.G. Altman, C. Gamble and P.R. Williamson. 2011. 'Frequency and Reasons for Outcome Reporting Bias in Clinical Trials: Interviews with Trialists', *British Medical Journal* 342, 10.1136/bmj.c7153.

Steinbrook, R. 2008. 'Saying No isn't NICE - The Travails of Britain's National Institute for Health and Clinical Excellence', *New England Journal of Medicine* 359(19), 1977–1981.

Stern, B.J. 1968. *Social Factors in Medical Progress*. New York: AMS Press.

Stewart, D.O. and J.P. DeMarco. 2005. 'An Economic Theory of Patient Decision Making', *Journal of Bioethical Inquiry* 2(3), 153–64.

Streefland, P. 2001. 'Public Doubts About Vaccination Safety and Resistance Against Vaccination', *Health Policy* 55, 159–72.

Sturdy, S. 2002a. 'Alternative Politics: The Development of Government Policy on Personal Health Care, 1905–11', in S. Sturdy (ed.), *Medicine, Health and the Public Sphere in Britain, 1600–2000*. London and New York: Routledge, pp. 241–59.

——— 2002b. 'Introduction', in S. Sturdy (ed.), *Medicine, Health and the Public Sphere in Britain, 1600–2000*. London and New York: Routledge, pp. 1–24.

Susser, M. 1998. 'Does Risk Factor Epidemiology Put Epidemiology at Risk? Peering into the Future', *Journal of Epidemiology and Community Health* 52, 608–11.

Szreter, S. 1995. 'The Importance of Social Intervention in Britain's Mortality Decline c.1850–1914: A Re-interpretation of the Role of Public Health', in B. Davey, A. Gray and C. Seale (eds), *Health and Disease: A Reader* (2nd edition). Buckingham: Open University Press, pp. 191–99.

Taylor, P. 2007. 'The Lay Contribution to Public Health', in J. Orme, J. Powell, P. Taylor and M. Grey (eds), *Public Health for the 21st Century: New Perspectives on Policy, Participation and Practice*. Maidenhead: Open University Press, pp. 98–117.

Taylor, S. and C. Ashworth. 1987. 'Durkheim and Social Realism: An Approach to Health and Illness', in G. Scambler (ed.), *Sociological Theory and Medical Sociology*. London: Tavistock, pp. 37–58.

Tenbensel, T. 2000. 'Health Prioritisation as Rationalist Policy Making: Problems, Prognoses and Prospects', *Policy and Politics* 28(3), 425–40.

Thompson, K. 1982. *Emile Durkheim*. London: Tavistock.

Thomson, G. and N. Wilson. 1997. *A Brief History of Tobacco Control in New Zealand*. Wellington: Australasian Faculty of Public Health Medicine (NZ).

——— 1999. 'Tobacco Control in New Zealand from 1945 to 1961', *New Zealand Medical Journal* 112, 101–3.

Tobias, M., T. Blakely, D. Matheson, K. Rasanathan and J. Atkinson. 2009. 'Changing Trends in Indigenous Inequalities in Mortality: Lessons from New Zealand', *International Journal of Epidemiology* 38, 1711–22.

Tombs, S. and D. Whyte. 2003. 'Scrutinizing the Powerful: Crime, Contemporary Political Economy, and Critical Social Research', in S. Tombs and D. Whyte (eds), *Unmasking the Crimes of the Powerful: Scrutinizing States and Corporations*. New York: Peter Lang, pp. 3–45.

——— 2007. *Safety Crimes*. Cullompton, Devon: Willan.

Tudor Hart, J. 2000. 'Commentary: Three Decades of the Inverse Care Law', *British Medical Journal* 7226, 18–19.

Turner, K. 1989. 'Safety, Discipline and the Manager: Building a "Higher Class of Men"', *Sociology* 33(4), 611–28.

van Netten, C., K. Teschke, V. Leung, Y. Chow and K. Bartlett. 2000. 'The Measurement of Volatile Constituents in Foray 48B, an Insecticide Prepared from Bacillus Thuringiensis Var. Kurstaki', *The Science of the Total Environment* 263(1–3), 155–60.

Vernon, J.G. 2003. 'Immunisation Policy: From Compliance to Concordance?', *British Journal of General Practice* 53, 399–404.

Watson, N. 2007. 'Disability and Public Health: From Resistance to Empowerment', in A. Scriven and S. Garman (eds), *Public Health: Social Context and Action*. Maidenhead: McGraw Hill/Open University Press, pp. 86–94.

Watterson, A. 1994. 'Whither Lay Epidemiology in UK Public Health Policy and Practice? Some Reflections on Occupational and Environmental Health Opportunities', *Journal of Public Health* 16(3), 270–74.

——— 1999. 'Why We Still Have "Old" Epidemics and "Endemics" in Occupational Health: Policy and Practice Failures and Some Possible Solutions', in N. Daykin and L. Doyal (eds), *Health and Work: Critical Perspectives*. Basingstoke: Macmillan, pp. 107–26.

Watts, G. 2006. 'Looking to the Future (1996)', in R. Porter (ed.), *The Cambridge History of Medicine*. Cambridge: Cambridge University Press, pp. 298–329.

Weindling, P. 2008. 'American Foundations and the Internationalizing of Public Health', in S. Gross Solomon, L. Murard and P. Zylberman (eds), *Shifting Boundaries of Public Health: Europe in the Twentieth Century*. Rochester: University of Rochester Press, pp. 63–86.

Weiss, A. 1993. 'Causal Stories, Scientific Information, and the Ozone Depletion Controversy: Intrusive Scenarios in the Policy Process', in T. Brante, S. Fuller and W. Lynch (eds), *Controversial Science: From Content to Contention*. Albany: State University of New York Press, pp. 225–40.

Westley, F. 1978. 'The Cult of Man: Durkheim's Predictions and New Religious Movements', *Sociological Analysis* 39, 135–45.

White, K. 1999. 'The Social Origins of Illness and the Development of the Sociology of Health', in C. Grbich (ed.), *Health in Australia: Sociological Concepts and Issues* (2nd edition). New South Wales: Longman, pp. 35–52.

Whiteis, D.G. 2008. 'Poverty, Policy and Pathogenesis: Economic Justice and Public Health in the U.S.A.', in J. Green and R. Labonté (eds), *Critical Perspectives in Public Health*. Abingdon and New York: Routledge, pp. 66–78.

Whitley, R. and K. McKenzie. 2005. 'Social Capital and Psychiatry: Review of the Literature', *Harvard Review of Psychiatry* 13, 71–84.

Wildavsky, A. and K. Drake. 1990. 'Theories of Risk Perception: Who Fears What and Why', *Daedalus* 119, 41–60.

Willis, K. 1999. 'Feminist Public Health Practice and Population-based Health Strategies: Breast Cancer Screening in Australia', *Scandinavian Journal of Public Health* 27(4), 245–46.

Wills, J. and A. Hales. 2005. 'Threads of Labour in the Global Garment Industry', in A. Hales and J. Wills (eds), *Threads of Labour: Garment Industry Supply Chains from the Workers' Perspective*. Oxford: Blackwell, pp. 1–15.

Wilson, M. 1992. 'Towards a Feminist Jurisprudence in Aotearoa', in R. Du Plessis (ed.), *Feminist Voices: Women's Studies Texts for Aotearoa/New Zealand*. Auckland: Oxford University Press, pp. 266–77.

Wood, P. 2005. *Dirt: Filth and Decay in a New World Arcadia*. Auckland: Auckland University Press.

Wooffitt, R. 2005. *Conversation Analysis and Discourse Analysis: A Comparative and Critical Introduction*. London: Sage.

World Health Organization 1986. *Ottawa Charter on Health Promotion*. Copenhagen: WHO Regional Office for Europe.

——— 2006. *World Health Report 2006: Working Together for Health*. Geneva: World Health Organization.

World Health Organization Regional Office for Europe 1985. *Targets for Health for All*. Copenhagen: World Health Organization.

Wynne, B. 1987. *Risk Management and Hazardous Waste: Implementation and the Dialectics of Credibility*. Berlin: Springer-Verlag.

——— 1989. 'Sheepfarming after Chernobyl: A Case Study in Communicating Scientific Information', *Environment* 31(2), 10–39.

——— 1995. 'Public Understanding of Science', in S. Jasanoff, G. Markle, J. Peterson and T. Pinch (eds), *Handbook of Science and Technology Studies.* Thousand Oaks, CA: Sage, pp. 361–88.

——— 1996. 'Misunderstood Misunderstandings: Social Identity and Public Uptake of Science', in A. Irwin and B. Wynne (eds), *Misunderstanding Science? The Public Reconstruction of Science and Technology.* Cambridge: Cambridge University Press, pp. 19–46.

Zierler, S. and N. Krieger. 2008. 'HIV Infection in Women: Social Inequalities as Determinants of Risk', in J. Green and R. Labonté (eds), *Critical Perspectives in Public Health.* Abingdon and New York: Routledge, pp. 47–65.

Zylberman, P. 2008. 'A Transatlantic Dispute: The Etiology of Malaria and the Redesign of the Mediterranean Landscape', in S. Gross Solomon, L. Murard and P. Zylberman (eds), *Shifting Boundaries of Public Health: Europe in the Twentieth Century.* Rochester: University of Rochester Press, pp. 269–97.

Index